Human Resource Development
Theories & Practices

Human Resource Development
Theories & Practices

Edited by

Harish Chandra

AKANSHA PUBLISHING HOUSE
NEW DELHI - 110 002 (INDIA)

AKANSHA PUBLISHING HOUSE
4649/21-B, Ansari Road,
Daryaganj, New Delhi - 110 002
Phones: 23263193, 9811582579
E-mail: ektabooks@yahoo.com

Human Resource Development: Theories & Practices

First Published, 2006

ISBN 81-8370-013-6

PRINTED IN INDIA

Published by M.P. Misra for Akansha Publishing House, New Delhi - 110 002 and Printed at Tarun Offset Press, Delhi

To
All Great Management Wizards
who have propounded the theories
for making HRD a success.

CONTENTS

Preface ix

1. Strategic Human Resource Development 1

2. Issues in Training and Employment 24

3. Human Resource Development: A Philosophical Interpretation 35

4. Concepts of Human Resource Planning 81

5. Human Resources Development Planning 104

6. HRD: Training and Development 113

7. Concept of Manpower Information Systems 130

8. Human Resource Flow Management 147

9. Managing Human Resources in Practice 197

10. Human Resource Management 237

Select Bibliography 260

Index 275

PREFACE

Recognition of 'Human Capital' or 'Human Resource' is rather a new phenomenon in arena of Development. Earlier in the process of production it was termed as 'Labour.' The early development planners over-emphasised the role of physical capital in economic growth. However the development literature of the 1950s and 1960s paid ample attention to the role of human beings as human capital, and by 1970s it recognised the development of human resources as the most crucial objective.

During the late nineteenth and first half of twentieth century, when the requirement for the workers in the developed countries, particularly in the United States of America was at its peak, the need for mass education to equip people with the requisite traits was felt. The emergence of opinion in favour of mass education and pervasive growth of "educational industry" in United States of America during this period was in a way a reflection of the scale at which industrial development required trained human resources.

The process continued during the early period of the twentieth century. It can be said that it came to its full, around the World War II. It is in this phase of industrial growth the linkages between education and employment, reached its climax. Consequently in the fifties, educational sector got recognised as a critical component of the growth process. The realisation led to the discovery of "human factor" and development analysis heralded the human capital revolution. Schultz, Harbison, Meyers and Becker led the parade which opened up several new areas of economic analysis including health, welfare, poverty and home economics.

Human Resource Development, has taken centre stage in the development debate. This is not one day too early, since the human condition and what can be done to improve it are close to the objectives of development than are the means and material requisites which have long been the preoccupation of economic development planners and policy-makers.

Human resources development (HRD) is the process of increasing the knowledge, the skills, and the capacities of all the people in the society. In economic terms, it could be described as the accumulation of human capital and its effective investment in the development of an economy. In political terms, human resource development prepares people for adult participation in political processes. From the social and cultural points of view, the development of human resources helps people lead fuller and affluent lives.

The concept of HRD has two facets—first, dealing with human resource development and second, with regard to its utilisation. There are several inputs which are required for the development and utilisation of human resources. For example, nutrition, drinking water, health, education, training, sports, culture, housing and communication etc. may be considered as critical for a proper development of these resources. Keeping in view the long gestation period that is required before the investment in human resources can start bearing fruit, it is necessary to have a continued commitment for the purpose.

Human resources are developed in many ways i.e., through formal-education, on-the-job training, self development, improvement of health and nutrition. HRD related activities seek to design, redesign and continuously upgrade the potential of human resources so that the latter continues to contribute to the process of development in a productive manner. This has to be so irrespective of the stage of economic growth and any particular phase through which the economy may be passing. It requires a detailed exercise in which the specificities of the society are especially taken note of. Thus, planning and management of human resources becomes a perennial exercise.

Many common supportive and trade-off linkages are there among the different components which go into the making of human resources. Hence it requires an integrated approach and one has to take a holistic view of the conditions under which human resources are suppored to be developing. More importantly, it is also clear that the combinations of these inputs may vary from period to period or from one situation to another.

Though plenty of standard literature is available on the subject and consequent upon further researches, new theories and practices come in as such HRD and HRM are developing day by day.

In this book, we have chosen some vital and crucial issues pertaining to the subject. Sources of information are secondary i.e., books, journals, abstracts, magazines etc. In fact the information is based on the theories, developed and propounded by various management experts, professionals and thinkers. As such entire credit for this venture goes to all those scholars whose opinions and works are liberally borrowed here. To make the book more comprehensive case studies, made by some scholars are also included.

We owe a deep sense of gratitude to all those great men of letters as well as the editors and copyright holders on whose painstaking researches, this book is devised. We are also grateful to different libraries for making available the requisite information. We are equally thankful to all those who have inspired and assisted us in one way or other. I am deeply beholden to my teachers and colleagues for guidance and moral support. Finally, I am thankful to my publisher Mr. M.P. Misra for bringing out this book.

I will feel amply rewarded if this work could help those for whom this is meant. Constructive criticisms and suggestions for improvement of quality of information are cordially invited from all quarters.

—*Editor*

1

STRATEGIC HUMAN RESOURCE DEVELOPMENT

> "A man who does not think and plan long ahead will find trouble right at his door."
>
> —*Confucius*

Strategic human resource development (SHRD) offers a proactive, value-adding, holistic, synergistic, and long-term perspective for "people-development" function in all forms of organisations. The basic philosophy is to help all employees recognise and realise their full potential as human beings, so that individuals, teams, and organisations can achieve their objectives both effectively and efficiently. SHRD can play a critical transformative role in the people resources.

Though Human Resource Development (HRD) is a relatively new term, but certainly not a new concept. The original roots of HRD can be traced directly to the earliest form of training, often referred to as vocational education, provided by the apprenticeship system in colonial America in the eighteenth century. With the advent of the industrial revolution during the late 1800s, the resultant factory system of production made it possible to increase production by using machines and unskilled workers. Eventually, many factories created 'factory schools' to train the engineers, machinists, and skilled mechanics who were needed in large numbers to design, build, and repair machines. During World War I many factories producing non-military goods had to retool their machinery and retrain their workers to meet a huge demand for military equipment. By the end of the nineteenth century, Taylor's (1911) principles of scientific management stressed the managerial responsibility of job design, selection, training, and planning. Factories started training more and more employees in the art of "one best way" to do a job. The human relations movement ignited by the Hawthorne Studies (1924-1932) of Elton Mayo and his associates broadened the scope of inquiry to the importance of human behaviour on the job (Mayo, 1933). The 1950sand 60s period can be considered as the true historical starting point of HRD and it is because of the behavioural science movement that HRD has had such a dramatic impact on modern organisations.

In the United States of America the first professional association focusing exclusively on HRD issues was founded in 1942 as the American Society for Training Directors. In 1945 the association published the first issue of *Industrial Training News*, renamed in 1947 the *Journal of Industrial Training*. In 1964 the association changed its name to the American Society for Training and Development (ASTD) owing to the realisation of a wider role and relevance of the professional trainers in such areas of employee development as coaching, counselling, and problem solving. During the late 1980s, the ASTD sponsored a two-year study to explore emerging models and to identify the HRD roles and competencies needed for an effective HRD function. The Models sought to provide tools that are detailed enough to reflect the vast differences in the organisation of HRD content, but at the same time they sought to develop a common language about HRD so that people can communicate about it, recognise similarities across jobs and train and educate others for HRD work. The Academy of Human Resource Development (AHRD) was established in the early 1990s by a group of HRD academics and it emerged as a significant source of scholarly literature on

HRD in the US. Gradually, many colleges and universities introduced HRD programmes in one of three academic departments: business/management, psychology, and education.

In the Great Britain the development of career professionals came somewhat later. It was triggered by the Industrial Training Act 1964 which introduced a network of Industrial Training Boards for designated industries, and a compulsory training levy/training grant system for all but small organisations (Walton 1999). It led in the same year to the formation of the Institute of Training Officers which in the late 1970s was renamed the Institute of Training and Development. In 1994, the Institute of Training and Development merged with the Institute of Personnel Management to form the Institute of Personnel and Development, currently known as Chartered Institute of Personnel and Development (CIPD).

The National Council for Vocational Qualifications (NCVQ) was set up in 1986 – a landmark development in the creation of the present national VET system in the UK. This led to the development of National Vocational Qualifications (NVQs) in England and Wales, and Scottish Vocational Qualifications (SVQs) in Scotland. The introduction of the NVQ system offered Britain for the first time in its history a structure of occupational qualifications comprising agreed national standards of competence across every recognised occupational area.

In the UK, HRD courses are more recent with the first professionally recognised HRD Master's programme being validated at South Bank University, London in 1991. The University Forum for HRD was established in 1992 as a national network of higher education institutions offering Master's degree in HRD, and the first UK professor in HRD was established at Liverpool John Moores University in 1993. In 1993 the university of Twente, the Netherlands coordinated a pan-European survey of HRD professionals and their practice by replicating the ASTD's study. The essential difference is that the ASTD study focused on future idealistic profiles, while the practitioner study in Europe focused on current HRD practices.

Historically, the development of HRD can be traced from training and instructional design, to training and development, to employee development, to human resource development. Perhaps the main advance of HRD as a field of academic study has taken roots in the USA pioneered initially by the ASTD, and taken further forward by its academic offshoot – the Academy of Human Resource Development (AHRD). New technology, globalisation, drive for quality, cost containment, market volatility, workforce diversity, the importance of knowledge capital, and the speed of change acted as the precursors of SHRD in progressive and result-oriented organisations of both developed and developing economies. These trends posed both challenge and opportunity for organisations to earn and sustain competitive advantage through developing multi-skilled, flexible, and committed workforces. While all nations have systems of workforce development and workplace learning and exhibit an amazing range of differences in their purposes, values, policies, structures, stakeholders, and patterns of participation, the UK and US are probably the two western nations where systems of HRD are most clearly identifiable, including academic preparation, professional certification, and formal acceptance of HRD roles in virtually all sectors of the world of work (Kuchinke,2002).

HRD: Theoretical Framework

Some of the prominent theory-building efforts of HRD scholars include—Systems Theory Applied to Human Resource Development (Jacobs, 1989), Foundations of Performance Improvement and Implications for Practice (Swanson 1999), A Theory of Intellectual Capital (Harris, 2000).

(i) General Systems Theory: This theory, the unit of analysis is understood as a complex of interdependent parts. An open (vs. closed) system is dependent on the environment for inputs, which are transformed during throughput to produce outputs that are exchanged in the environment. According to a competence management model of organisations, skills and abilities are treated as inputs from the environment; employee behaviours are treated as throughput; and employee satisfaction and performance are treated as outputs.

(ii) Human Capital Theory: Human capital refers to the productive capabilities of people. Skills, experience, and knowledge have economic value to organisations because they enable it to be productive and adaptable; thus, people constitute the organisations's human capital. All costs related to eliciting productive behaviours from employees constitute human capital investments made in anticipation of future returns.

(iii) Institutional Theory: Institutional theory views organisations as social entities that seek approval for their performances in socially constructed environments. Organisations conform to gain legitimacy and acceptance, which facilitate survival. Because multiple constituencies control needed resources, legitimacy and acceptance are sought from many stakeholders. Studies on institutionalisation focuses on pressures emanating from the internal (formalised structures and processes, informal or emergent group and organisation processes) and external (government laws and regulations, licensure and certification of profession, and existing practices within the industry) environments.

(iv) Resource-Based Theory: This theory of the firm blends concepts from organisational economics and strategic management. A basic assumption of this view is that organisations can be successful if they gain and maintain

competitive advantage. Competitive advantage is gained by implementing a value-creating strategy that competitors cannot easily copy and sustain and for which there are no ready substitutes. Three types of resources available to organisations are (a) physical (plant, technology and equipment, geographic location), (b) human (employees' experience and knowledge), and (c) organisational (structure; systems for planning, monitoring, and controlling activities; social relations within the organisation and between the organisation and external constituencies).

Human Resource Development

The most fundamental basic elements associated with the concept of HRD are education, training, development, and learning. Whereas *Education* is defined as 'activities which aim to develop the knowledge, skills, moral values and understanding required in all aspects of life rather than a knowledge and skill relating to only a limited field of activity. The basic purpose of education is to develop in an integrated way an individual's intellectual capability (training the mind), conceptual and social understanding, and work performance.

While *'Training'* is learning that is provided in order to improve performance of an individual to improve performance in the present job. Training is a planned process to modify attitude, knowledge or skill behaviour through learning experience to achieve effective performance in an activity or range of activities. Its purpose, in the work situation, is to develop the abilities of the individual and satisfy the current and future needs of the organisation.

The term "development" is used to denote learning experiences of any kind, whereby individuals and groups acquire enhanced knowledge, skills, values or behaviour. Its outcomes unfold through time, rather than immediately, and they tend to be long-lasting.'

Whereas *'Learning'* is 'a relatively permanent change in behaviour that occurs as a result of practice or experience' and it refers to the process of unlearning what has been wrongly learnt over the years, relearning new things which are relevant for the current and future needs, and getting oneself committed to the continuous process of learning and development.

Originally, human resource development was conceived as a composite term incorporating three types of vocational learning activity that would contribute to making individuals more effective at work: (a) training, focusing on immediate changes in job performance; (b) education, geared towards intermediate changes in individual capabilities; and (c) development concerned with long-term improvement in the individual worker. In response to the changing HRD practice, Nadler reformulated HRD in 1989 as 'organised learning experiences provided for employees within a specified period of time to bring about the possibility of performance improvement and/or personal growth'.

In this connection McLean and McLean (2001:322) expressed ggested the following integrated view:

> Human resource development is any process or activity that, either initially or over the long term, has the potential to develop adults' work-based knowledge, expertise, productivity and satisfaction, whether for personal or group/team gain, or for the benefit of an organisation, community, nation or, ultimately, the whole of humanity.

Megginson et al. (1993) consider HRD as an 'integrated and holistic approach to changing work related behaviour, using a range of learning techniques and strategies.' As the strategic significance of organisational learning as a source of competitive advantage gains recognition, a strategic need arises for appropriately positioned 'learning architects' with the distinctive competencies to orchestrate learning initiatives on behalf of organisations (University Forum for HRD, 1995).

The hallmark of HRD is, a deliberate focus on 'learning' (intentional or accidental). Stewart (1998) differentiates between 'learning' and 'interventions,' which he considers to be two distinct processes contributing to HRD. 'Learning' can, will, and does happen, irrespective of the wishes or actions of anyone. It is as natural and inevitable as breathing. However, the practice of HRD is constituted by deliberate, purposive, and active 'interventions' in the natural process of learning. Such interventions can take many forms, most capable of categorising as education or training or development.

Now, a transformative approach to HRD allows it to be complementary to the conventional Human resource management, rather than relegating it as to a subservient role. McLagan (1989) uses a human resource wheel to portray the distinctive role of HRD in relation to the human resource management, i.e. its focus on the 'development' issues – 'training and development,' organisation 'development,' and career 'development.' Selection and staffing, performance management systems, human resource planning, and organisation/job design are the HRM areas. Which are linked as a set of processes for achieving a set of strategic results such as productivity, quality, innovation, human resource fulfilment, and readiness for change.

Strategic Human Resource Development (SHRD)

Strategic human resource development (SHRD) refers to 'development that arises from a clear vision about people's abilities and potential, and operates within the overall strategic framework of the business. SHRD puts particular emphasis on the development of comprehensive, coordinated and dynamic approaches for major learning initiatives within and outside an organisation in order to facilitate the achievement of corporate objectives in a competitive environment (University Forum for HRD, 1995).

Traditionally HRD is preoccupied with designing and delivering training and development programmes, and at times, it runs the danger of adopting a piecemeal approach to the overall development of the individuals, teams and organisation without an explicit coherence among its strategies and activities on the one hand and, on the other, an absence of vertical linkage and alignment with the business strategy and organisational vision. According to Walton, SHRD brings a transformative focus to the HRD with its holistic orchestration of learning within organisations.

In SHRD, people development and the supporting learning processes are one of the strategic capabilities and distinctive competences of those organisations that effectively undertake them. Learning and development initiatives are undertaken with full strategic intent, with an understanding of how they add to the coherence of the knowledge creation, development, and application at levels in the organisation, congruent with an explicit learning philosophy incorporated into the overall organisational vision and mission. Similarly, education, training, and development initiatives are undertaken with an explicit strategic intent and with the total commitment and involvement of those people who are supposed to benefit from them. SHRD is a strategically important partner assuming the same level of importance as the traditional core organisational processes: financc, production, and marketing. SHRD is concerned with the management of employee learning for the long-term, keeping in mind the explicit corporate and business strategies. It genuinely establishes strategic partnerships across the organisational spectrum ranging from influencing people development policy decisions at the board level to effectively collaborating with line managers and other personnel practitioners. Further it ensures that there exists an organisational strategy for the HRD effort that guides, unifies, and provides direction to 'planned learning' sponsored by the organisation. Men at all levels in the organisation's chain of command willingly share responsibility and accountability for HRD. Thus, SHRD demonstrably contributes to the long-term survival, growth, and excellence of the organisation by ensuring a favourable learning climate and encouraging the employees to challenge the status quo through innovation, change, and continuous learning and development.

Main Features of SHRD

1. *External Environment Analysis:* SHRD function builds capacity to analyse and understand the external environment.

2. *Business-led Approach:* SHRD function strives for constant alignment with the mission, goals and the genuine needs of the organisation.

3. *Top Management Support, Involvement, and Commitment:* SHRD function cannot be integrated into strategy unless senior managers want that to happen. The extent to which SHRD becomes a feature of strategy, therefore, largely depends on the ability and willingness of top managers to visualise important environmental trends in SHRD terms.

4. *As Formal Policy Statement:* SHRD policy statement serves many purposes such as guiding management in the identification and implementation of appropriate and relevant SHRD activities; spreading awareness among supervisors, line managers, and top managers about their individual and collective SHRD responsibilities on a regular basis; communicating to everyone why the organisation is investing in various SHRD programmes; defining the relationship between the organisational objectives and its commitment to

the SHRD function; helping continually to assess the learning needs and providing a framework for evaluating SHRD programmes.

5. *Integration of HRD and HRM activities:* A strategic approach to HRD is fundamental to the adoption of a comprehensive human resource management approach in the organisation. Not only does SHRD provide an impetus for a more integrated HRM approach, but it is also necessary to have a close integration between HRD and other HRM activities.

6. *Enthusing Line Manager:* The line manager is best placed to assess, on an ongoing basis, the training and development needs of subordinates, and can facilitate in identifying development routes for subordinates and is ideally placed to offer advice, direction, and counselling to subordinates. Several research studies pointed out the competency deficiencies of line managers in such areas as inability to appraise performance, lack of counselling skills, inability to identify skill gaps, poor listening skills, and inability to empathise with their subordinates.

7. *Marketing:* For the SHRD policy to work, it must be known, understood, and accepted by those implementing it and affected by it. To make this happen, HRD specialists should be good at marketing their services by educating and convincing the top management and line managers about the potential contribution of SHRD.

8. *Context-specific:* The philosophy, policies, processes, programmes, and practices of SHRD are influenced by a host of factors shaping and reshaping the internal and external environments of organisations. The internal contextual factors include technology, structure, size, life-cycle stages, existing and required competencies of individuals and teams, and business strategy. The external contextual factors are legal,

social, and political environments; unionisation; labour market conditions; industry characteristics; and national cultures. The legal, social, and political environments are bound to impact SHRD initiatives. The union-management relations within each firm may be adversarial or cooperative, which in turn may influence the successful implementation of various SHRD initiatives. This increasing workforce diversity has clear implications for training, development, and mentoring. SHRD is country-specific and cross-national differences can be noticed in the way in which SHRD policies and programmes are being evolved and implemented.

9. ***Stakeholder-driven approach:*** Within the context of SHRD, a stakeholder is anyone whose actions can affect the management of SHRD activities within the organisation. Key stakeholders include: top management, line managers, training and development specialists, personnel managers/HR specialists, individual employees, external training providers, educational establishments, and trade unions. Stakeholders may have different values and expectations which will influence their reaction to various learning and development initiatives undertaken by the organisation. SHRD calls for a symbiotic and synergistic approach ensuring commonality of interests; mutual trust, confidence and goodwill; and a shared vision among the key stakeholders for the successful implementation of training, education, and development programmes.

10. ***Evaluation:*** Strategically-oriented HRD functions invest time, energy, and resources in evaluating their activities and they use measures that seem most relevant to the management of their own organisation (Zenger and Hurgis,1982; Stewart,1999). SHRD also advocates that managers, supervisors, and employees should be evaluated on how well they develop themselves and contribute to the development of others in the organisation.

11. ***Corporate Strategy and Culture:*** A strategic HRD function must be matched with the corporate strategy and culture. It has to establish options, policies, and plans that fit the strategic logic and cultural web found in the organisation (Edwards and Kleiner,1988; Denison,1984).

12. ***Wider Applicability:*** SHRD Principles are applicable to any conceivable organisation - private, public, or MNE; for-profit or not for-profit; voluntary or employing - where people are found working together in groups for the effective and efficient accomplishment of organisational goals.

13. ***Large Scope:*** SHRD can be viewed as a proactive, system-wide intervention linked to strategic planning and cultural change. On the contrary, the traditional view of training and development consists of reactive, piecemeal interventions in response to specific problems. SHRD advocates the involvement of many stakeholders such as supervisors, line managers, human resource colleagues, training and development specialists and top management rather than simply the training and development function acting as a provider.

SHRD can influence and also be influenced by the national and global developments (macro) in the field. Human capital, conceptualised as a stock of skills and knowledge, is perhaps a significant factor explaining the differential rates of economic growth of nations. SHRD, with its focus on humans, is heavily influenced by the context in which it is studied and practised.

Notably, global human resource development takes place across more than one culture or nation, and may occur on an international (between nations), multinational (many nations), and regional (e.g., Asian, European, Pacific Rim, Latin America) scale. Although global SHRD involves the same practice areas, roles, functions, and activities of domestic SHRD, it is shaped and reshaped by several factors such as the composition of the trainees, cultural differences among trainers and trainees, and physical and financial resources available to the global SHRD practitioner.

Training and Development

An appropriate, suitable and adequate provision of training and development may contribute to the organisational progress in many ways. First, a more highly skilled workforce may increase productivity by producing a higher level of output or by producing output of greater value. While, a well-trained and motivated workforce may cut the costs of supervision, as they possess the skills to inspect their own work and become self-managed. Again, a skilled workforce can also improve the firm's functional flexibility since they are much easier to retrain owing to their relatively broad knowledge-base and multi-skills. Further, a technically competent workforce can also give management confidence in utilising new technology and provide employers with more scope for rapid adjustment in production methods, product requirements and technology. The management's commitment to training and developing the employees in an attempt to improve product quality and service delivery bears a symbolic significance in that it sends a signal to the workforce that they are valued in the organisation.

The benefits of training and development can be realised only through the systematic implementation of employee training and management development policies and programmes. It is not enough to believe in training as an act of faith. This belief must be supported by a positive and realistic philosophy of how training contributes to the bottom line. Training and development should not be treated as an expenditure, but it needs to be clearly demonstrated that it is an investment which would pay rich dividends in the long run. The systems approach to planned training is underpinning this belief and it consists of the following five inter-linked steps: identifying training needs, defining learning requirements, planning training programmes, implementing training, and evaluating training evaluation.

Career Development

Career development is an organised, planned effort comprised of structured activities or processes that result in a mutual career plotting effort between employees and the organisation. Within this system, the employee is responsible for career planning and the organisation is responsible for career management (Gutteridge and Otte,1983). According to Sachein, such planning needs to be appreciated that the relationship that binds individual and organisation is two-fold: legal contract (specifying duties, terms and conditions, and material rewards) and psychological contract (felt and perceived expectations, wants and rights). The challenge is one of matching the needs of the organisation with those of the people who work for it, and to do so from entry into the organisation, through each career transition-point thereafter, until exit, in order to achieve a mutually beneficial relationship over time.

It is increasingly recognised that today employees are operating in an age of discontinuity – either they are holding temporarily permanent or permanently temporary jobs. In this context of unstable employment environments, employees will not be able to make decisions and take action that will ensure continuous work life with a single employer. The traditional concept of 'career' is now replaced by 'portfolio' of transferable skills and competences, and new ideas and understandings of careers place much more weight on the active agency of individuals. There is a breakdown in the 'old deal' of job security, a fair day's pay, and career development in return for loyalty, commitment and, at least, a fair day's work. Instead, they are being offered a 'new deal' involving less security but the chance to make themselves more employable in the future.

Today's employees are becoming more concerned than ever with keeping their skills, abilities, and knowledge current, and preparing for tomorrow's new tasks. As far as career development function is concerned, the individual employee is responsible for maintaining his or her employability and marketability both within and outside the organisation. On the other hand, the employer's responsibility is limited to providing support for employees to continually add to their skills, abilities, and knowledge creating growth opportunities, financial assistance, and providing the time for employees to learn. Many organisations are now offering opportunities for individuals to develop their skills and competencies to increase their marketability or employability.

Organisational Development

Organisational development (OD) is basically the process of enhancing the effectiveness of an organisation and the well-being of its members through planned interventions that apply behavioural science concepts and is a system-wide process of data collection, diagnosis, action planning, intervention, and evaluation aimed at: (1) enhancing congruence between organisational structure, process, strategy, people, and culture; (2) developing new and creative organisational solutions; and (3) developing the organisation's self-renewing capacity (Beer 1983).

Techniques

Some of the OD techniques or interventions aimed at bringing about planned change include: sensitivity training (training groups that seek to change behaviour through unstructured group interaction); survey feedback (the use of questionnaires to identify discrepancies among member perceptions, discussion follows and remedies are suggested);

process consultation (consultant gives a client insights into what is going on around the client, within the client, and between the client and other people, and identifies processes that need improvement); teambuilding (high interaction among team members to increase trust and openness); and inter-group development (OD efforts to change the attitudes, stereotypes, and perceptions that groups have of each other).

Learning

As a highly complex human process, 'learning' incompasses the acquisition of new or/and fine-tuning the existing knowledge, skills, attitudes, values, and habits. It encompasses individual, team, and organisational learning experiences triggered by failures, successes, and anything in between. Learning is, a continuous process, and 'learning to learn' is the most fundamental learning of all. Organisations do not perform the actions that produce the learning; it is individual members of the organisation who behave in ways that lead to it, although organisations can create conditions which facilitate such learning

Knowledge management is a relatively new but much debated in management research and practice. The increasing relevance and strategic significance of knowledge management in modern organisations are due to the continuous rise of technological opportunities (internet and intranet, e-learning), new competitors and new requests by customers, demand for proactive strategies aimed at continuously renewing the sources of competitive advantage. The emphasis on the knowledge management and development process progressively went from mere information and knowledge exchange to knowledge embodiment and transfer for re-use and, finally, to the overall process of knowledge creation, diffusion and refinement over time.

The development of knowledge is repeatedly claimed to

be an essential determinant of organisational profitability. In a knowledge economy, organisational success is largely hinging on the rapid generation and application of knowledge to achieve organisational objectives. People are becoming knowledge workers, expected to know more, learn more quickly and cope with ever more frequent change. Knowledge workers are individuals who have high levels of education and specialist skills combined with the ability to apply these skills to identify and solve organisational problems.

It is to be noted that SHRD practices associated with creating the right environment for sharing knowledge will in particular promote organisational learning by creating a 'rich landscape of learning and development opportunities'

The SHRD function should be able to effectively handle the challenges involved in successfully positioning and applying the management and development of knowledge within and across organisations such as the management of values and culture, providing clear direction to the people involved, ensuring aligned and measured processes to facilitate knowledge creation and development, encouraging the appropriate use of technology, obtaining collaboration and teamwork from knowledge workers.

Summing Up

Organisational success is heavily dependent upon a skilled, flexible, and highly motivated workforce that is geared towards achieving continuous improvement. Transformative HRD policies and practices of an organisation must be driven by the business strategy. Human resources can be integrated into strategic plans and the company's strategic plans are likely to be more successfully implemented only if HR policies cohere, if line managers have internalised the importance of human resources and this is reflected in their behaviour, and if employees identify with the company. Thus, SHRD is concerned with the provision of training, education, development, and learning opportunities for continuous transformative improvement in individual, team, and organisational performance.

There is a need to evolve a conceptually sound, analytically perfect, and operationally feasible model of SHRD reflecting ideological underpinnings and a holistic context. Closer and effective collaboration and interaction must be encouraged between HRD researchers and HRD practitioners in order to build more accurate empirical evidence of SHRD policies and practices in different types of organisations.

SHRD practitioners have to adopt a professional (expert and ethical) approach to the development of people at work. Efforts should be made to remove actual and potential barriers to the credibility and effectiveness of SHRD in organisations.

REFERENCES

Argyris, C. (1957). *Personality and organisation.* New York: Harper & Row.

Ashton, D. (1984). Current issues in line/staff relationships. *Management Education & Development*, 10(2): 105-18.

Baird,L.,Meshoulam,I. (1988). Managing the two fits of strategic human resource management. *Academy of Management Review*,13: 116-28.

Barney, J. (1991). Firm resources and sustained competitive advantage. *Journal of Management*,17: 99-120.

Becker, G.S. (1964). *Human Capital.* New York: National Bureau of Economic Research.

Beer, M. (1983). What is organisational development?. In: Baird, L.S., Schneier, C.E. and Laird, D. Eds. *Training and development sourcebook.* Amherst, MA: HRD Press.

Beer, M. and Spector, B. (1989). Corporate wide transformations in human resource management. In: Walton, R.E. and Lawrence, P.R. Eds. *Human resource management: Trends and challenges.* Boston, MA: Harvard University School Press.

Bennet, R (1988). The nature and context of training for success. *Journal of European Industrial Training*, 12(2): 3-7.

Brewster, C., Hegewisch, A., Lockhart, T. and Holden,L. Eds. (1993). *The European human resource management guide*. New York: Academic.

Brown, G. and Read, A.R. (1984). Personnel and training policies – Some lessons for western companies. *Long Range Planning*, 17(2): 48-57.

Burgoyne, J. (1988). Management development for the individual and the organisation. *Personnel Management*, June: 40-44.

Child, J. (1977). *Organisation*. New York: Harper & Row.

Conner, K.R. (1991). A historical perspective of resource-based theory and five schools of thought within industrial organisation economics: Do we need a new theory of the firm?. *Journal of Management*, 17: 121-54.

Drucker, P. (1993). *Post-capitalist society*. Oxford: Butterworth-Heinemann.

Ferris, G.R., Buckley, M.R., and Allen, G.M. (1992). Promotion systems in organisations. *Human Resource Planning*, 15: 47-68.

Flamholtz, E.G., and Lacey, J.M. (1981). *Personnel management, human capital theory, and human resource accounting*. Los Angeles: Institute of Industrial Relations, University of California.

Garrat, R. (1990). *Creating a learning organisation*. London: Institute of Directors.

Garvin, D.A. (1993). Building a learning organisation. *Harvard Business Review*, July-August: 78-91.

Grant, R.M. (1991). The resource-based theory of competitive advantage: Implications for strategy formulation. *California Management Review*, 33(3):114-135.

Greenhaus, J.H. (1987). *Career Management*. New York: Dryden Press.

Guest, D.E. (1991). Personnel management: The end of orthodoxy. *British Journal of Industrial Relations*, 29(2): 149-76.

Gunningle, P and Flood, P. (1990). *Personnel management in Ireland: Practice, trends and developments*. Dublin: Gill & Macmillan.

Gutteridge, T.G. and Otte, F.L. (1983). *Organisational career development: State of the practice*. Washington, DC: ASTD Press.

Hall, D.T. (1984). Human resource development and organisational effectiveness. In: Fombrun, C.J., Tichy, N.M. and Devanna, M.A. Eds. *Strategic human resource management*. New York: John Wiley and Sons, 159-81.

Harris, L. (2000). A theory of intellectual capital. In: R.W.Herling and Provo, J. Eds. *Strategic perspectives on knowledge, competence, and expertise*. San Francisco: Berrett-Koehler: 22-37.

Harrison, R. (1997). *Employee development*. London: Institute of Personnel and Development.

Herriot, P. (1992). *The career management challenge. Balancing individual and organisational needs*. London: Sage.

Higgs, M. (1989). A strategic approach to training and development. *Training and Development*, November: 11-14.

Honey, P. (1998). The debate starts here. *People Management*, 1 October: 28-29.

Hoyle, E. (1995). The school as a learning organisation. *Paper delivered at the AERA Conference*, San Francisco, April.

Huber, G. (1991). Organisational learning: The contributing processes and literatures. *Organisation Science*, February: 88-115.

Jacobs, R.L. (1989). Systems theory applied to human resource development. In:

Johnson, G. and Scholes, K. (1997). *Exploring corporate strategy*, 4th edition, Hemel Hempstead: Prentice-Hall.

Kim, D.H. (1993). The link between individual and organisational learning. *Sloan Management Review*, Fall: 37-50.

Kuchinke, P.K. (2002). Comparing national systems of human resource development: Role and function of post-baccalaureate HRD courses of study in the UK and US. *Third conference on HRD research and practice across Europe, Edinburgh, 25-26 January, 2002.*

Likert, R. (1961). *New patterns of management*. New York: Harper & Row.

Mankin, D.P. (2001). A model for human resource development. *Human Resource Development International*, 4(1): 66-85.

Marsick, V.J. (1994). Trends in managerial invention: Creating a learning map. *Management Learning*, 21(1): 11-33.

Mayo, E. (1933). *The human problems of an industrial civilization*. New York: Macmillan.

McGoldrick, J. and Stewart, J. Ed. (1996). *Human resource development: Perspectives, strategies and practice*. London: Pitman.

McGoldrick, J., Stewart, J and Watson, S. Eds. (2002). *Understanding human resource development: A research-based approach*. London: Routledge.

McLagan, P.A. (1983). *Models for excellence: The conclusions and recommendations of the ASTD training and development competency study*. Washington, DC: ASTD.

McLagan, P.A. and D.Suhadolnick. (1989). *Models for HRD practice: The research report*. Alexandria, VA: American Society for Training and Development.

McLean, G.N. and McLean, L. (2001), If we can't define HRD in one country, how can we define it in an international context. *Human Resource Development International*, 4(3): 313-26.

Meyer, J.W., and Rowan, B. (1977). Institutionalised organisations: Formal structure as myth and ceremony. *American Journal of Sociology*, 83: 340-63.

Miller, P (1987). Strategic industrial relations and human resource management: Distinction, definition, and recognition. *Journal of Management Studies*, 24: 101-109.

Mumford, A. (1989). *Management development: Strategies for action*. London: Kogan Page.

Nadler, L. (1970). *Developing human resources*. Houston: Gulf.

Nonaka, I. (1991). The knowledge-creating company. Harvard Business Review, November-December: 96-104.

Ouchi, W.G. (1981). *Theory Z: How American business can meet the Japanese challenge*. Reading, MA: Addison-Wesley.

Peters, T. and Waterman, R. (1982). *In search of excellence*. New York: Harper & Row.

Phatak, A.V. (1992). *International dimensions of management*. Boston: PWS-Kent.

Powell, G.N., and Butterfield, D.A. (1994). Investigating the "glass ceiling" phenomenon: An empirical study of actual promotions to top management. *Academy of Management Journal*, 37: 68-96.

Reid, M.A. and Barrington, H. (1997). *Training interventions: Managing employee development*. 5th edition. London: Institute of Personnel and Development.

Schein, E.H. (1978). *Career dynamics: Matching individual and organisational needs*. Reading, MA: Addison-Wesley.

Scott, W.R. (1987). The adolescence of institutional theory. *Administrative Science Quarterly*, 32: 493-511.

Senge, P. (1990). *The fifth discipline: The art and practice of the learning organisation*. London: Century Business.

Stead, V and Lee, M. (1996). Inter-cultural perspectives on HRD. In:

J.Stewart and J.McGoldrick. Eds. *Human resource development: Perspectives, strategies and practice.* London: Pitman, 47-70.

Stewart, J. and Tansley, C. (2002). *Training in the knowledge based economy.* London: CIPD.

Stewart, J. (1996). *Managing change through training and development*. 2nd edition. London: Kogan Page.

Streeck, W. (1989). Skills and the limits of neo-liberalism: The enterprise of the future as a place of learning. *Work, Employment and Society*, 3(1): 90-104.

Swanson, R.A., (2001). Human resource development and its underlying theory. *Human Resource Development International*, 4(3): 299-312.

Taylor, F.W. (1911). *Principles of scientific management*. New York: Harper.

Trist, E and Bamforth, K. (1951). Some social and psychological consequences of the longwall method of coal-getting. *Human Relations*, 4: 3-38.

University Forum for Human Resource Development (1995). *Emerging concept of HRD – A position statement*. London: UFHRD.

Walton, J. (1999). *Strategic human resource development*. Essex: Financial Times/Prentice Hall.

Wenger, E. and Snyder, W.M. (2000). Communities of practice: The organisational frontier. *Harvard Business Review*, January-February: 33-41.

Wilson, J. Ed. (1999). *Human resource development*. London: Kogan Page.

Yadapadithaya, P.S. (2000). Training and development in India. *International Journal of Training and Development*, International Briefing 5, 4(1): 79-89.

Zenger, J. (1985). Training for organisational excellence. Journal of European Industrial Training, 9(7): 3-8.

2

ISSUES IN TRAINING AND EMPLOYMENT

"Undertake something that is difficult; it will do you good. Unless you try to do something beyond what you have already mastered, you will never grow." —*Ronald E. Osborn*

While the global current economic transition offers tremendous opportunities for organizations to gain competitive advantage based on their distinctive competencies, it also brings with it certain threats to the identity and continued survival of various organized sectors of human activity. Seemingly, the near demise of public sector undertakings, growing incidence of acquisition and merger, arrival of MNC's, growing and potential sickness of several productive and service sectors coupled with unbalanced economic growth, rising consumerism and ever increasing unemployment have created uncertainties of a magnitude that Indian society is confronting for the first time.

Apparently the impact of these changes has been most felt amongst the employees in both the organized and unorganized sectors of the economy. The pressure generated by the environment to transform a 'low performance – high cost' economy to 'high performance – low cost' economy will lead organizations to adopt the approach of downsizing of resources resulting in surplus manpower which will add to the already swelling pool of unemployed and underemployed workforce in the country. By doing so they would have created for themselves a social environment which will be unstable, hostile and volcanic. It is in the backdrop of this scenario that organizations have to generate options to ensure their sustenance and growth without sacrificing the goodwill of the people directly or indirectly engaged in contributing to their existence as producers of wealth and providers of services. Organizations will have to develop active adaptive strategies and coping mechanisms to respond to the changes within and outside their boundaries.

In a rapidly changing environment, the pace and direction of adaptation best suited to the individual organization is not easily identifiable. The task of anticipating and getting an organization to move towards change, cannot be accomplished by one person. The difficulty arises on account of non-compliance, resistance and growing alienation not only among the workmen but also the middle ranks of management. The problems that organizations will face, therefore, relate to cost and effort needed to introduce change, gain acceptance for it and coping with its unanticipated consequences. Management of change, thus, must become the major thrust and preoccupation of HRD efforts.

HRD cannot be looked at as an activity separate from the challenges being encountered by organizations and their requisite responses to those challenges. HRD effort must inextricably be linked with strategic thinking and organization design and development efforts. The relationship among the three is interactive and dynamic characterized by directive correlation. The interrelationship among strategic planning, organization design and manpower development constitutes a major and perhaps a fundamental shift in the way organizations of the future will respond to environmental changes and justify their raison d'etre by meeting demands for which they were created. Developing appropriate designs of organization will be the key factor in providing competitive edge in the global market.

Emerging Priorities

The Human Resource Development Strategies must reflect the following:

1. Developing employees competence enabling them to equip broad range of skills, more relevant knowledge and increased autonomy and discretion.
2. Awareness of the total system of production/service so that exigencies of the task requirements, changing priorities and variation standards can be responded to promptly.
3. Appreciation of the products and services flow in the market place and dynamic and interactive relationship with various stakeholders such as changing customer needs and expectations, suppliers and contractors etc.
4. Skills to manage heterogeneous teams of workers in such a way as to create synergistic effect and to communicate internally with speed and clarity.
5. Increasing concerns over job security and career growth necessitating large investments in retraining and employability.
6. Regular improvement in productivity of resources and quality of product at par with global standards.
7. Sustaining and creating a culture of excellence with balanced stress on organizational effectiveness, quality of life and social accountability.
8. Strategic planning as a centralized activity loses much of its relevance. It is the process of planning itself that allows employee to develop alternative scenarios, articulate or validate their beliefs and assumptions and act as flexible guides for the future.
9. Planning for organizational revitalization, morale building, participatory management for mutuality of

influence and individual revitalization though continuing education programmes.

Strategic HRD

The nature and extent of influence exercised by employees in the affairs of the an organisaiton tends to vary from one organization to another. The trend, however, seems to be in the direction of enlarging the areas of employees' influence particularly in matters relating to their work, their careers, and personnel policies affecting their morale and commitment.

Yet another area where policies need to be formulated, concerns inflow and outflow of employees. The trend seems to be towards attracting and retaining talented and skilled manpower. As such the selection process, needs to be designed tact for both the potential member and the organization so that they are able to enter into a longer term psychological contract through need alignment and goal congruence.

Career growth would need to be redefined in terms of lateral and cross-functional movement of employees. Further, career growth prospects will have to be measured in terms of job content and skill requirement rather than in terms of status or position in the hierarchy of an organization. The area and extent of vertical and horizontal specialization necessitated by the nature of technology and strategic considerations will be decided by the organization as career paths available to its employees. Thus, status will be delinked from the nature of job leading to situations where movement could be even downward.

Again, competitive and fast changing environment necessitates cutting down fats through downsizing resulting in threat to job security at middle, supervisory and workmen level. Organizations, however, do make use of multiple criteria for retention of employees in the face of imminent redundancy.

Performance may not be the sole criterion; employee commitment and loyalty, impact of economic cycles on employment stability, social obligations, political compulsions, etc. are other criteria used in decision for retention. Considering the unemployment situation in the country and availability of trained manpower in traditional skills, organizations do have the option of laying off surplus human resources. If at all, lay off becomes inevitable, it is desirable to openly communicate and involve the concerned groups and their representatives so that various options are explored and the decision will thus acquire more acceptability.

With the qualitative change in the nature of workforce who are professionally and technically trained, organization is viewed not as a source of supplementary income but as an instrument for growth and development of one's professional expertise and enhancement of one's quality of life. Consequently there has been a shift in emphasis from 'monetary reward' to 'intrinsic rewards' like responsibility, self fulfillment, social status, etc. The reward systems will have to be flexible enough to attract and retain employees, reinforce learning and competence, encourage multiskilling and cross-functional expertise acquisition, inculcate team spirit and enhance collective performance, ensure long term viability and health of the system, and achieve need alignment through active participation.

Work system is an area, that must become the central core around which HRD strategies and policies should be devised. One-man-one job as the basic building block of the organization leads to elongated hierarchical levels, elaborated horizontal differentiation, compartmentalized operations along functions and authority levels resulting in increased decision response time, high costs of coordination and control, pressures for vertical movement, and limits realization and utilization of human potentialities. Human resource development efforts do not always lead to enhanced organization success due to the nature of the design of the work system.

There is a world wide movement to organize work around integrated teams, diagonal teams, problem solving groups, productivity improvement groups, quality circles and the like to create learning organizations capable of responding with speed to the challenges of change and thus enabling organizations to maintain their competitive edge. Together with the shift towards team management and advancement in and adoption of information technology, managerial and supervisory levels are progressively being reduced.

Human resource is an asset and it is the management's responsibility to ensure their effective utilization and development by creating avenues and opportunities that the environment offers. Obviously, Training and retraining activities, can prevent the occurrence of a crisis situation leading to retrenchment of the employees. Organizations both public and private – find themselves in this situation as they could not apparently anticipate changes and formulate plans to manage the change. Search for establishing linkages between the current and future requirements of the organization and manpower training needs must become an on-going process.

Development efforts through training or continuing education programmes need to be integrated into the work system so that they contribute to enhanced organizational effectiveness and increased personal efficacy.

Training

The training activities, to contribute meaningfully to the success of an organization, should take into consideration the following:

1. The purpose of training and priorities of goals to be achieved through training will obviously depend on strategic

options of corporations. Strategic considerations like, expansion, diversification, single product – single market, etc. would determine the direction of the training and development effort. The divisions, units, departments or work groups may widely differ on strategic goals in the same corporation.

2. The cultural factors like concern for employees comfort and welfare, commitment to internal development, dedication to social/community, responsibility, power and status differentiation in the organization will have influence in determining the direction the training and development effort might take.

3. The contextual factors such as sectoral changes, competitive threats, economic fluctuations, technological advancements and rising aspirations of workforce for career growth will also have implications for prioritization of various training needs.

Types of Training Activities

I. Task-Skill Training

(i) Acquisition

(ii) Socialization of new entrants

(iii) Developing such an advanced skills not easily available in the labour market

(iv) Changing job responsibilities for assigned position

(v) Improving job quality and productivity.

II. Career Advancement

(i) Attracting and retaining talent

(ii) Retraining dislocated manpower

(iii) Providing skills to advancing managers

(iv) Reinvigorating exhausted workers

(v) Assisting the exit process - pre retirement counseling, out placement, etc.

III. Organizational Effectiveness

(i) Improving work-group effectiveness

(ii) Reinforcing a company culture and core values

(iii) Changing an existing culture and inculcating new values.

(iv) Rewarding performance or long service

(v) Enriching the work experience of workers

IV. Interface Effectiveness

(i) Changing customers/user group's needs and expectations

(ii) Meeting various statutory/non statutory requirements

(iii) Conflicting demands of the stakeholders and strategies / tactics for reconciliations

(iv) Supplier/vendor development

(v) Entrepreneurial orientations and skill for the community/society

In keeping with the kind of scenario that is emerging, the thrust areas for training and retraining are likely to be the following:

1. Multi-Skilling

Multiskilling, in addition to harnessing of untapped potentials of the employees, provides flexibility in deployment of human resources to meet the exigencies of the work system. At managerial level, cross-functional training will assume far greater importance for ensuring speedy decisions with broader perspective, introducing innovations, and for reduction in the cost of co-ordination and control. Horizontal mobility at all levels in the organization will become an important issue for success of organization.

2. *Customer Orientation*

In fact there is already a visible trend to restructure organizations based on the concept of internal customer to enable the work groups orient their efforts and output for meeting their specifications and priorities. Customer satisfaction is a concern that has, by and large, been neglected by most organizations in India. In the changing scenario, customer orientation will hold the key for success of organizations regardless of their business interests.

3. *Team Management*

The teams provide the mechanism for achieving high level of vertical and horizontal integration and creating synergy. Managing through team serves the twin purposes of enhancing task excellence as well as contributing to the development of its members.

4. *Out Placement*

As a strategy to deal with surplus employees, a number of organizations in the U.S. and Europe, have begun to provide training in marketable skills and provide assistance in finding employment elsewhere sometimes even outside the industry. This sort of assistance is also being provided to managerial and supervisory staff who are to be laid off. The measures to encourage employees to look for alternative employment often include free training, reimbursement of expenses for attending interview calls.

5. *Quality and Productivity*

Productivity and quality of products and services have already been recognized as a major thrust area for training by most organizations in India for gaining and retaining competitive advantage in national and global markets. Productivity and quality improvement programmes must get the utmost priority over any other activities in the context of existing and emergent global scenario. Increasing number of organizations has qualified for certification in quality in terms of international standards. Training in quality circles, and productivity improvement techniques are already being conducted in a large number of organizations with the help of external as well as in house trainers and facilitators.

6. *Empowerment*

To get best out of people and to elicit their willing support to organization's endeavour, the employees must be made to feel powerful, a mental and psychic state of being in command, releasing and using one's energy in productive pursuits and actively influencing and transforming situation conducive to achievement of one's goals and purposes. The workmen, their representatives and the managerial staff need to be given training in empowerment so that they are encouraged to make productive use of their potential power.

7. *Entrepreneurship*

Entrepreneurial training will enable employees to manage their respective work groups as an entrepreneurial venture and small business, to take risks in trying out new ideas and be accountable for their decisions. The skills acquired through training can also be utilized by employees in taking up subcontracting from the organization, setting up ancillary firms or establishing trade or business of their own.

8. *Perspective Building*

Perspective building and enlarging the perceptual map of the employee at all levels incorporating various interest groups will increasingly become a major thrust area of training to enable them to think globally. The changes in the structure of organizations and their response patterns to transforming realities of the world of business must be accompanied by corresponding changes in employees' perceptual map and perspective through which they comprehend, understand

and interpret the world around them and select appropriate and adaptive responses.

REFERENCES

- Burton, Cary and Anton Frankeiss, (1994), *Training for Total Quality Management*, Gower Publishing Ltd.
- Kleiman, Lawrence S., (2003), *Human Resource Management – A Managerial Tool for Competitive Advantage* (3rd Edn.), Published by Biztantra, New Delhi.
- Wexley, Kenneth, N. and Gary P. Latham, (2002), *Developing and Training Human Resources in Organizations*, 3rd Edition, Prentice Hall, New Jersey.

3

HUMAN RESOURCE DEVELOPMENT: A PHILOSOPHICAL INTERPRETATION

> "Every man is to be respected as an absolute end in himself; and it is a crime against the dignity that belong to him as a human being to use him as a mere means for some esternal purpose."
>
> —*Immanuel Kant*

The evolutions of agricultural, cultural, industrial, social, and economic developments in their natural courses have witnessed various changes in the sphere of human behaviour, custom, values and also in the working conditions of people engaged in different professions. It has further been observed that the pattern of life at its different stages has always tried to invite affluence. With the passage of time, a tendency towards the formation of an affluent society has been developed among people.

The formation of such affluent society has again resulted into the creation of various classes of demands, particularly in the areas of obtaining various services towards satisfaction. This sort of observation has been well-explained in Maslow's analysis of need. The development of industrial economy possibly speaks of the greater need for more service to the people. The gradual increasing demand for more services to the people has ultimately given rise to the necessity for larger production and better services to the people.

But, as always, production is a function of a combination of inputs—men, material and money. In a similar manner, services are also the functions of human beings and many other associated inputs. All these indicate that of the various resources usually employed in the different development processes, human resource is assumed to be the most important and unlimited one. It is probably a more important aspect of achievement than any smooth and effective direction of things to be done. The only thing is that such a resource always needs a little bit of orientation.

Effectiveness and Measurement

The human resource is assumed to be a source of innovation for improvement in modern technology, skill and their effective utilisation. Therefore it can be presumed that in the process of development, any investment in human resource is likely to be more effective even in the utilisation of material capital. The utility of all human beings can be viewed from their family perspectives, social values and organisational uses. The value of such a resource to each class of individuals changes with the change in the quality, of the resource and its utility to each sector of the society or business environment. In that context, therefore, it is both static as well as dynamic. It is static when there is neither any improvement nor any deterioration in the quality of such resource.

Again, it is dynamic when there is a definite improvement in the quality of such a resource. However, the value of such a resource cannot possibly be measured in quantitative terms, although there has been a constant, effort to give strees to quantitative approach to the problem during these days. The basic ingredient in the development process, especially in the areas of economic and social development, is probably human resource, the acquisition and formation of capital being only secondary to exploitation of 'human brain'. An integration of skill and ability of human beings has therefore been considered as the controlling key to a balanced economic performance and development. In that context, human resource development is always a function of proper utilisation of creative opportunities and available environment through acquisition of knowledge, skill and incentives, usually necessary for productive efforts. The said productive efforts become still more meaningful when they are tagged with other inputs like material and machine. In reality, the effort of inputs like men, materials and machines have a multiplier effect, the result of which is usually received as return against the cost incurred for human capital. This may be one of the reasons why human resource cannot be measured independently. That is, the economic value of the people at work cannot possibly be measured in terms of money. The fundamental issues that can be raised here are that the human value, human behaviour, human action, human thoughts, human characteristics—all these qualities cannot in any case be measured in terms of money, possibly for the facts that such qualities are always subject to constant fluctuations according to the conditions or circumstances prevailing at a certain point of time.

Thus the quality of life in all spheres, be it in working life, family life, social or cultural life, is likely to be changed according to the mental make-up and physical capabilities of the individuals at a specific point of time. Therefore any attempt to account for certain classes of human resource, i. e., management staff, technical personnel, skilled workers etc., in their respective money value is likely to be turned into a futile exercise. Human resource, in reality, is always considered to be above everything, not to speak of money. But for proper allocation of such resources and also for their optimum uses, it can, at best, be assessed in qualitative terms. As outputs are always the functions of input-mix, therefore the contribution made to that effect by human beings towards achieving the ultimate object of improving human welfare, cannot in any case be segregated merely to evaluate that in quantitative term. It may be pointed out in that context that knowledge, intellect, experience and even physical strength—all are usually utilised in boosting up the moral, social, cultural and economic upliftment of human beings. They are all invested either for production and distribution or for consumption and satisfaction, possibly with the object of maximising human welfare. Under the circumstances, any misconception of measuring the said resources in quantitative term is expected to be ruled out at the outset.

Organisational Perspective

An organisation is ordinarily considered to be the most essential unit when its employees are usually given the scope for personal growth, preferably with high ethical and moral standard. They are expected to be given that scope, objectively with equality of opportunity to all of them. The employees in their turn also are to equip themselves by improving their capabilities through acquisition of knowledge and experience. A noble attempt towards that end is likely to help them to develop excellence among themselves. The process of development thus started is likely to be continued throughout their lives. The organisation in its turn is also expected to assess the entire stock of human resources available to it, probably for allocation and optimum uses of such resources. The entire stock that is assessed may finally be suitably channelised into various productive efforts through different logical decisions and creative actions. But an organisation is able to acquire excellence for productive efforts only when it abides by the law of human engineering—the system of proportions. We know that all human beings are normally to follow certain laws for conservation of their energies. Thus the law of conservation of energy appears to have applied to all human beings. The principle of homeostasis tells us that the different organs usually have the tendency to co-operate among themselves. They usually follow a specific system to maintain a regular equilibrium in the entire body mechanism. That is why we normally observe that the body mechanism has always a tendency to have an energy balance. As a result, energy intake in the body tends to be equal to energy output. A biological rythm is assumed to have taken place in the body of all human beings. With that concept in view, the concept of homeostasis has subsequently been developed. That concept obviously helps to find out or locate the behaviouristic pattern of each and every individual, primarily in the light of various motivational factors. The homeostasis, in fact, is a circular feedback; regulation process. It symbolises that the maintenance of an equilibrium stage through control of the variables is the only way to achieve one's desired goal. As against that another theory of identical but of refined nature has been propounded which is known as the theory of open systems.

Unlike the homeostasis which merely decides the principles of primary needs of human beings for survival and self-preservation, the open systems speak of growth and expansion. In economic and business organisations generally two categories of human resources are observed—internal human resources and external human resources. The internal human resources consist of staff employed in an organisation and the external human resources comprised of customers, creditors, shareholders and public in general. But whatever may be the categories of such resources, they can always be developed through knowledge, experience and well-directed physical effort. The ultimate objective is surely to promote human welfare.

Again, as a result of the development of human resources, three types of variables are usually observed—casual, intervening and end result variables. The casual variables are changes in subordinate attitudes. The intervening variables on the other hand are the functions of confidence, trust, attitudes, subordinate leadership behaviour and group processes. The end result variables are the functions of scrap, productivity, satisfaction of different parties and groups performance of effectiveness etc. Unfortunately, all those variables may not always move in the same direction. Under the circumstances, the effectiveness of the human resource development programme may only be perceived through an application of a series of experimental parameters. Thus the effectiveness of a training programme can be judged on the basis of the power of receptivity, communication effectiveness and the environment. The power of receptivity is again dependent on the motivation of the employees. The scope of application of the feedback principle to improve relationship also determine the magnitude of effectiveness of the available human resources of an organisation. Then again, the system approach, in decision-making, application of communication, human relations approach, the qualifications and experiences of the existing staff having specific aptitude in business—all will probably speak of the specific model of the human resources development programme pattern of an organisation. The leadership style in management could therefore be 'accordingly fixed-up. Now, it appears that the journey towards effectiveness to a large extent is likely to be blocked if human resources of an organisation cannot be suitably developed according to the necessity of the circumstances.

The differences in the level of performances are possibly the functions of abilities and motives of the individuals. This has pointedly been elaborated by Victor H. Vroom. Our experience in the past shows that the effect of ability and motivation on performances always interact with each other. Thus it shows that the effect of motivation on performance is dependent on the level of ability of a worker and further the impact of ability on performance is contingent on the motivation of a worker. According to Victor H. Vroom, this multiplicative relationship can be presented as:

$$\text{Performance} = f(\text{Ability} \times \text{Motivation})$$

Any fluctuation in the value of one is certainly to influence the performance capability of an individual. In the light of any expansion programme or diversification or adoption of new technology, the manpower planning in an organisation is expected to be done on the basis of the specific need of the organisation concerned. For specific industry, however, such a planning technique is likely to cover through manpower forecasting. In a similar manner, sectorwise, the manpower need for any specific sector like agricultural sector or industrial sector or service sector is to be assessed with due caution and care. At the national level, however, such a planning process is to be effected on the basis of the national plans and programmes for development activities. In that connection, it may be stressed here that. the occupational distribution and the factor-like the mobility of labour are always to be taken into account.

The need for a systematic discipline to develop various categories of people, is specially pressing in the developing countries like India. The ability to equip people, however, will depend on the capability of the individuals on one hand and the scope for adopting a particular discipline that can be taught to those individuals on the other. To enter into an area of knowledge utility is possibly the right step towards self-development. It helps to acquire information which, in fact, may act as energy for developing various types of mental aptitude for all human beings. The human beings are to acquire knowledge informations, mainly to preserve that for future use. Those informations will be of immense use as aids to the field of teaching and learning. But the pace of human resource development is not likely to reach to its optimum stage unless along with normal teaching and learning processess through intensive studies, research and experiences, people from all walks of life are allowed to think and analyse the pros and cons of the implications of those informations.

In that connection, it may be pointed out that self-consciousness and consciousness in the performance of duties are also to be established within oneslf. One must also be sincere in one's effort to perform a specific job and for that one is also expected to assess one's capability. In fact, all people must have certain definite and positive policies according to the suitability of a particular environmental situation.

The human resource developmental science in a like manner is expected to develop in itself an appropriate logistic approach. Any attempt to raise human intellect to the required standard is therefore likely to follow a series of concerted and planned actions. Again, even if such actions are taken in time, in that case also it becomes difficult to preserve human resource development process continuously. In reality, human resource preservation is possibly the greatest difficulty that men are facing today. The present day socio-economic changes that are taking place due to changes in the environmental conditions, particularly with respect to dynamic economic developmental activities in the sphere of industrial growth, have resulted in constant changes in human behaviour, attitude, perception etc. Due to constant pressure of population, there has also been considerable stake on the preservation of human resources. This is particularly true not only in the case of measurement through quantitative parameters but also in terms of qualitative dimensions. A massive and coordinated effort having a sustained effect will be the right direction for any substantial change to that effect.

To achieve excellence in any field, one is certainly to gain academic excellence and experience in the concerned field. But any environmental condition prejudicial to the development of excellence is not likely to help to bring out best in people. It is to be remembered in that context that the adoption of a particular technique is not normally an end in itself. To reach at the optimum developmental stage, one is surely to realise the effectiveness of each individual course of action.

Philosophy of Management: An Introduction

The term management has been defined by different people in different ways—some have defined it in a simple way and some in a complex way. Management means the manner in which a given task is executed and supervised. It also implies accomplishing a task within limited resources available and the skill in the manipulation of the resources.

Management is often viewed according to one's way of thinking. To a design engineer it may mean a matter of designing products, utilities and, equipment. To a techno-economist or a cost accountant it may appear to be a matter of figures that can spell in monetary terms either loss or gain. To a research chemist it may mean formulaes, chemical reactions and processes.

The fault lies not with these individuals but with the environment in which they have grown up and with the organisations that keep them in isolation and do not acquaint them with the various facts of management. Unconsciously, a technical bias of the work being done by them sets into their sub-conscious mind. This is due primarily to the fact that no one has guided them as to what management actually means. Such people, when they rise to high positions by virtue of their long years of experience, find themselves in a difficult situation because of their technological bias and low professional standards. Owing to their lack of far-sightedness and initiative, they fail to grasp the essentials of various other disciplines around them.

Since management is responsible for getting the assigned task done within the given time, the given resources and in a particular manner, an acceptable definition, to our way of things, could be: "Management is getting things done through people by effective *utilisation of resources, time and environment"*. Resources include government policies, legal frameworks, economic and social factors, competition, etc.

WHAT MANAGEMENT DOES?

We shall try to reason out and assess as to what management does rather than quote some readily available definitions to make the meaning of the term management explicit.

For example, let us determine the work that is involved in the construction of a mini steel plant. What are the major elements of work involved in it? Broadly, these are:

(i) Preparation of a feasibility report;

(ii) working out a detailed project report;

(iii) projection of time schedule or pert network for completion of the project;

(iv) arrangement and allocation of funds;

(v) selection of personnel and procurement of equipment;

(vi) erection;

(vii) commissioning; and

(viii) despatch, marketing, finance and other commercial aspects.

FUNCTIONS OF MANAGEMENT

If we break these broad items into finer elements and analyse the nature of work involved in each of them, the process will reveal five basic elements which go into management. These are:

(1) Planning the course of action to be adopted to attain predetermined objectives;

(2) setting up an organisational structure and assigning specific responsibilities to different individuals;

(3) directing and coordinating the efforts of all members working for the organisation;

(4) controlling the activities of the members through setting up standards for their performance;

(5) motivating the members to cooperate with one another for the achievement of the objectives.

Planning

Planning aims at achieving the desired results. It entails advance thinking of events to come, such as organisation, allocation of resources, framing of policies, setting of objectives, purchase of raw-materials, and other items; storage, marketing; fixing of time schedules for construction, provisioning of matching facilities etc. It would naturally include preparation of broad guidelines, that would help in the execution of the work within the available resources, in time, and subject to the existing restraints, the industrial policies of the State and the social responsibilities of business.

Organisation

The second fundamental element may be defined as determining the activities necessary for executing a plan of action and assigning such activities to groups of individuals. The organisational structure so set up is the framework within which the total proceeds of executive control is carried on. This fact emphasises the importance of a sound organisational structure.

Coordiantion

Coordination seeks to blend the available factors into a relationship so that the plan can be put into effect. Modern business has a multitude of inter-dependent operations.

Balancing the work and efforts of individuals into those of a group, and allocation and adjustment of resources are delicate functions. The efforts of many disciplines have to be harmonised for synchronised action. The task of blending the activities of different individuals, groups, machineries, processes and maintaining the inter-dependence of operations as well as reconciling their differences is done by coordination.

Control

It ensures that the activities are executed in terms of the plan. It includes follow-up. Determining a plan of action is not the end. Constant follow-up has to be maintained to see the job through. For this, it is necessary to provide an organisation or establishment with a formal line of authority which would be responsible for organisation, follow-up and control, outline strategies to make up for the loss either in units of time or quantum of production; check the plans as projected against the actual status at a point of time; measure the performance against the norms laid, record necessary statistical details for a comparison and basis of realistic planning for the future and taking corrective measures necessary to make the plan operative. Control is thus a continuous process of decision-making and embodying the decisions in the form of specific instructions on behalf of the management.

Motivation

Directions or orders alone cannot deliver the goods. The human mind has to be motivated to think and give of its best. Instilling a team spirit in the group and motivate them to be loyal, and obedient; making them aware of their sense of responsibility; and making them put their joint efforts are necessary for the fulfilment of the targets. Motivation is thus a process of inspiration that enable the members of the group to pull their weight effectively, to give group loyality and to jointly meet the challenge that the group has accepted.

These are called fundamental elements because the correctness and successful execution of managerial decisions depend upon the extent to which these elements have gone into the making and execution of these decisions.

In case all the above mentioned functions are carried out smoothly, the task is accomplished within the time schedule resources available and in the manner desired. However, in actual practice, this is not the case. Mistakes; wrong directives; lack of coordination; loss of opportunity; defective planning; communication gap; group frictions; misunderstanding; professional jealousy; etc., which are common to any organised activity, keep the task from being accomplished. These factors are also described as the forces of misdirection and activity trap in management terminology. External forces, which are outside the boundary of the organisation, also limit managerial effectiveness.

Management as such is the amalgam of the broad functions outlined above and many other sub-functions or specialist functions that are associated with it. Each aspect or each function is a part of the management and all have a contribution to make towards the total process.

Of the five principal functions of management discussed above, all are not technical; some are social functions as well. Management, therefore, is not only technical but also involves human factors and relations. Since it is chiefly the activities of the people that are to be coordinated and regulated by the management, it is also called a social or socio-technical process.

We may therefore deduce that management is a social process entailing responsibility for realistic planning, organisation, coordination; effective follow-up (control) and group motivation for the fulfilment of a given task or purpose.

Evolution of Management

To understand fully the intricacies of management, so far explained, it is necessary to indicate briefly the history and evolution of management.

Management has been of some concern to organised society throughout civilised history. Initially, contributions came from practitioners and later from theorists.

MANAGEMENT IN ANTIQUITY

Necessity and awareness of the need of management skills date back to the period beyond the beginning of recorded history. In the villages of the Euphrates Valley, priests who were worshipped by the people as representatives of God had evolved a system of management. Those priests had laid down rules for organising trade, the work of labourers societies, soldiers, etc. They employed men to keep records and prepare reports. The Indus Valley civilisation was an excellent example of planning and administration of township.

Similar records exist in the case of ancient China. Confucius' parables include practical suggestions for public administration and admonition to choose honest, sincere and dynamic officers. Records of early Greece do not give much insight into the principle of management. But the Athenian system of courts, administrative councils and board of generals indicated the existence of a system of managerial functions.

The history of the Roman Empire also gives much evidence of managerial knowledge in the fields of army operations and civilian/government administration. The Roman Catholic church also made notable contributions to organisation and management.

These principles of organisation and management were, somehow, lost sight of during the Dark Ages and up to the end of the sixteenth century. They had to be gradually rediscovered between the sixteenth and twentieth centuries. The history of this re-discovery can be traced through four different phases, viz.:

(i) a psychological process

(ii) an art

(iii) a systematic practice

(iv) a science.

MANAGEMENT AS A PSYCHOLOGICAL PROCESS

Entrepreneurs had neither any experience of their own nor of others to guide them in their work in the early days of the Industrial Revolution. They had, therefore, to depend entirely on their inborn abilities and skills in the performance of their job. This gave rise to the belief that management was basically a psychological process. Importance of qualities such as intuition and foresight gave further support to the belief that management flowed from certain inner impulses of individual managers. In short, it gave rise to a strong and universal belief that managers, poets and artists, were born and could not be made.

MANAGEMENT AS AN ART

There was, however, another school of thought which did not recognise or accept this view of management. They argued that if this view were correct, then superior managers could be developed simply by a strict adherence to the principles of the science of Eugenics. Actual experience had frequently shown that the successors of some distinguished founders and managers of industries were not so capable and occasionally were utter failures. This gave rise to the doubt that abilities to manage were not inborn. Acceptance of this theory helped to raise the status of management from a psychological process to that of an art.

MANAGEMENT AS SYSTEMATISED PRACTICE

Management was regarded as an art as long as practising managers were greatly engrossed in their day-to-day activities and had to depend on their personal abilities and skills to tackle their problems. In course of time, however, managers were able to observe some of their colleagues at work with whom they exchanged their views on mutual problems. Such exchanges enabled them to discard their old hit-or-miss method/practices and adopt those which had proved successful.

For quite some time, the practising managers did not consider it necessary to analyse the cause and effect relationship underlying such practices. They were content to adhere to them so long as they got satisfactory results. In this way, a large number of useful practices, DOs and Do NOTs came to be accumulated and the later generations of managers had no difficulty in adopting them. Management at this stage took to systematised practices of the past. However, this frequently resulted in a rigid and conservative attitude, since many managers who had found these practices successful refused to abandon them later when they had become out of date due to change of conditions.

MANAGEMENT AS A SCIENCE

This last and most important phase in the evolution of management was brought about by the operation of two forces: one, was the effort of practising managers to establish standard practices and, the other, the effort of scientists to demonstrate the application of the scientific methods of observation, experiment and verification in the field of management.

The first scientist to attempt this was Charles Babbage, a British mathematician. Having studied industry from outside, he came to the conclusion that the method of science could be applied to the operations in factories. He, therefore, recommended "accurate observation, exact measurement and precise knowledge of the cause and effect relationship as a substitute for guess work, intuition, and opinion."

It was, however, left to Frederik Winslow Taylor to synthesise and present as a reasonably coherent whole, ideas which had been a germinating force in Great Britain and the United States during the last few decades of the nineteenth century. He gave to a disconcerted series of initiatives and experiments a philosophy and a title. It was he who, for the first time, asserted that the study of management required adequate intelligence, an orderly habit of the mind and the ability to see a subject as a whole while keeping track of the parts. Since then, many others, notable among them being Henri Fayol, Mary Parker Follet, Elton Mayo, Chester I Bernard, L. Urwick, Doulgas McGregor, etc., have made very significant contributions to the theory of management and have helped to raise its status to that of science.

DEVELOPMENT OF THE THEORY OF MANAGEMENT

For about twenty years Taylor's book on scientific management was confined to applications in machine shops and factories. Simultaneously, his ideas were being developed and refined by Gilbreth, Emerson, Gantt and others. Still, it essentially dealt with the technical aspects of management. It was Henry Fayol who applied the same methods and techniques to the analysis of the work of a chief executive in a factory and thereby extended the scope of scientific management.

He was followed by Mooney Reiley, Chester I Bernard, L. Urwick, E.F.L. Breach who developed and refined the principles of administration formulated by Fayol. In spite of these developments, there were many who were sceptical about scientific management, because they felt that some important segment of management was missing from it.

It was left to Prof. Elton Mayo and Prof. Roethlisberger to discover this missing segment of human relations in management and to prove conclusively that attitudes of individuals and groups towards their work and towards one another have as much influence on the quantity and quality of their output as material and technical factors. This discovery opened a new vista to sociologists, research workers and thinkers, among whom Mary Parker Follett, L. Urwick and Douglas McGregor have received worldwide recognition for their valuable contributions.

F.W. Taylor

The honour of being the first to establish the claim of management as a science has been unanimously given to F.W. Taylor. His two important books on management are *Shop Management* published in 1903 and *Principles of Scientific Management* published in 1911. According to him, if a machine shop or a factory is to work with a reasonable degree of efficiency it must have the following five features:

(i) It must be organised on a functional basis so that the work of planning and of supervision is taken away from the departmental foreman and entrusted to those persons who are specialists in their own fields.

(ii) Various jobs must be carefully analysed with the help of the techniques of motion study, time study and fatigue study.

(iii) Machines and tools must be standardised.

(iv) The method of wage payment must be such as to provide adequate incentive to more efficient workers and penalty to the less efficient ones.

(v) There must be a complete mental revolution on the part of both the employers and the employees towards their work and towards each other.

The basics of Taylor's scheme of scientific management lie in functional organisation. Its central idea is the division of the work of management in a workshop, in such a way that each executive, from an assistant superintendent to a supervisor, has as few functions as possible to perform. Taylor sought to achieve this by setting up a planning department which would be responsible for planning all work, including work of a routine nature connected with planning.

Henri Fayol

Henri Fayol's book *The General and Industrial Administration* was, in large measure, a complement to Taylor's work. Fayol's book is divided into two parts: the first is concerned with the theory of administration and the second with training for administration. In the first part, he gives a classification of the main groups of operations to be found in any business.

He distinguishes six such groups, viz., technical, commercial, financial, security, accounting and administrative. The administrative group of operations is further classified into five sub-groups concerned with organisation, coordination, command, control, forecasting and planning.

He then points out that administration is not something set above the other operations, but is merely a specialised function which occurs in a greater or lesser degree in relation to all business activities. As one goes higher up the ladder of hierarchy, administrative knowledge and skill become relatively more important than technical skill.

According to him, it is the inability or unwillingness of the top executive to recognise this fact that is often responsible for the failure of a business.

Having analysed the nature of administration, Fayol listed fourteen principles which formed the core of his theory of administration. These are:

(i) Authority and responsibility;

(ii) discipline;

(iii) unity of command;

(iv) unity of direction;

(v) subordination of individual interest to general interest;

(vi) division of work;

(vii) remuneration to personnel;

(viii) centralisation;

(ix) scalar chain;

(x) order;

(xi) equity;

(xii) stability of tenure of personnel;

(xiii) initiative;

(xiv) *Esprit de Carps:*

These principles of administration were also accepted by L. Urwick and others as quite complete and comprehensive.

Having enumerated the principles of administration, Fayol went on to discuss the five elements of management, viz., planning, organisation, coordination, motivation and control which we have already discussed in the earlier part of this chapter.

Parker Follett

Miss Mary Parker Follet was the first to make managers and management thinkers of her time aware of the realities of human behaviour through her writings. Being intensely conscious of man's group life she saw that a person's association with his fellowmen gives rise to powerful emotions which colour his every action as a member of a group. He ceases to be the sole creator of his own thoughts and actions and comes to be moulded by the influence that the group exerts. A human group has, therefore, a life that is something more than the sum of the individual lives composing it. This philosophy of dominance of the emotions in human behaviour underlines all her analysis of the industrial organisation and its problems.

According to her, conflict in an organisation arises not out of difference of opinion between individuals but out of the failure of the individuals to make their differences contribute to the common cause. Another important concept in her analysis is the concept of authority which, as generally thought of in terms of status, is of one man having power over another. From her intimate study of human behaviour, Miss Follet pointed out that the personal subordination is offensive to human emotions and if it is made the foundation of an organisation, it may cause resentment and friction. To avoid these undesired reactions, she suggested that orders and authority must be depersonalised.

Prof. Elton Mayo

Prof Mayo was the first to get the opportunity of indicating the truth of the analysis of the behaviour of work groups. His experiments clearly demonstrated the tremendous influence of emotions on group behaviour. Through these experiments it was discovered that the rapid rise in the output of the test group was largely in response to an emotional stimulus. Many management thinkers tried to reappraise the prevailing management techniques in the light of the conclusions that were arrived at by Elton Mayo and his followers; among these, Chester I. Bernard and L. Urwick are the most well-known. Chester I. Bernard published his book *The Functions of the Executive in* 1939 and it has been said that this made as deep an impression as Taylor's *Shop Management* had done on the thinking of serious minded business leaders about the nature of their work.

As a result of all these developments, it is now being clearly realised by an increasing number of executives in business that, in addition to problems of the task, of adjustment of the individual to the task, and of arranging and correcting the tasks, there is an equally important problem of motivating the members of a group. This has naturally led to an increasing emphasis on such concepts as leadership, informal organisation and morale in the theory and practice of management today.

Douglas McGregor

Douglas McGregor challenged some of the prevailing concepts about the attitude of people towards work, and the system of reward and punishment to get things done. He described the traditional concept of management as theory X and the modern concept as theory Y. The traditional managers, according to him, emphasise on directing and controlling the efforts of others. They believe that man does not want to work, he shirks from responsibility, resists change, lacks ambition and is not very bright. Unless a system of reward and punishment is introduced, which would create fear in his mind, he will not work. The traditional approach thus rests upon the basic distrust of human nature.

The new theory of management, according to McGregor, looks upon man as a social being who likes work as much as rest or play. He wants to share the responsibility of and grow with the organisation. If people do not give of their best in an organisation it is not because of dislike for work or irresponsibility on their part, but because of the environment of the organisation in which they work. If management creates opportunities and permits people to be creative and responsible, they feel motivated. The carrot and stick policy, according to this theory, does not work. Instead, the principle of self-direction and self-control works better. Management in McGregor's view is thus "a process primarily of creating opportunities, releasing potential, removing obstacles, encouraging growth, providing guidance."

The application of new approach requires decentralisation and delegation of authority, job enlargement, participation and consultative management and self-evaluation in place of conventional performance appraisal by the supervisors. McGregor believes that only the management that has confidence in human capacities and is itself directed towards organisational objectives rather than towards the preservation of personal power can grasp the implications of this emerging theory.

LONG SHORT RANGE ACTIVITIES

The activities of management broadly can be depicted as follows:

The following functions, in actual practice, are very varied in nature and depend on the type of enterprise one is working in. These can be further divided into short-term or current functions and long-term or future functions.

The major short-term or day-to-day functions are:

- Production
- Quality Control
- Maintenance
- Personnel
- Finance and Accounting
- Marketing and Commercial
- Material Management

- Operations Research
- Stores and Purchase
- Public Relations
- and other allied aspects

The functions which come under the long-term or future field of activities are:

(i) Long-term policy decisions like whether diversify the activities or specialise in field of business; share of total market to be controlled.

(ii) Centralisation or de-centralisation of management.

(iii) Long-term planning and action needed. Suppose a steel plant of a capacity of 2.0 million tonnes per annum wants to attain a capacity of 10 million tonnes over a period of 15 years. It has to have a detailed plan to locate raw materials, machinery, spares, energy, finance, personnel and other infrastructures.

(iv) Research and development to consider the changes continually taking place in process, products, usage, technology, pricing, etc.

A future manager has to face many problems which managers in the past did not consider important. Such problems would arise because of changes like:

- Bigger business
- Individualism
- Less managerial authority
- Stronger unions
- Differential incentives
- Higher levels of education and specialisation
- Larger population

- Possible shorter shift durations
- Rapid technological changes
- Fewer operatives and more managers
- Community participations
- Government interference in favour of workers
- and many other allied factors.

A unified and integrated concept of management is therefore of prime importance. This would enable the manager to plan, sequence his work and delegate authority to appropriate hands/levels. Since the role of a manager is not to do each job himself but to get it done in a proper manner by inspiring, leading, driving, coordinating and directing the workers/executives to achieve the objectives of the management, he has to analyse his job, determine the interdependence of jobs and find out the extent to which he should do his work and distribute the work to be done by others. A manager will thus become more successful and effective if he successfully adopts the use of the unified concept of management.

GRADING THE MANAGEMENT

The form of the management hierarchy varies from country to country, depending upon social outlook, political cults and a number of other factors. However, the most common forms of management hierarchy are:

- Top management
- Middle management
- and specialists (Engineers, technologists, statisticians, etc.
- First line supervisors

Top Management

Top management is the key-stone in the arch of management. The top manager may be an owner, promoter or a professional manager. His function is to establish the conditions under which other members of the management can achieve their goals by performing the tasks assigned to them. The success of the organisation would depend upon the extent to which he can infuse the whole hierarchy in the management with energy, drive, vision and to the extent of effective communication between the members of the team.

Middle Management

Middle management plays a vital role in communicating the objectives and policies of the top management to the line supervisors. The middle managers are also responsible for feed-back from line supervisors to the top management.

Specialists

Specialists are organisational pillars on which rests the responsibility of maintenance of various professional skills and disciplines. They transform ideas into practice, analyse, suggest and improve technology, innovate, devise logistics and strategies for the growth/welfare of the organisation. By virtue of their skill and mental prowess they can be paid and placed in any of the management cadres depending on their educational background as well as their achievements.

Front-Line Supervisors

The line supervisors are responsible for conducting day-to-day operations of a company as per pre-determined schedules and also for achieving targets set up by the management. They maintain close contact with the workers and thus form an important link between the workers and the middle management.

HOW MANAGEMENT IS VIEWED

Management is often viewed or regarded as: (i) an economic resource, (ii) a system of authority , and (iii) a class or elite

(i) Economic Resource

The theory of management as an economic resource views management as a factor of production along with land, labour, capital and natural resources. The basic propositions which are fundamental to the understanding of management as an economic resource are:

Complexity of Business: Adequate managerial resources arc needed for complex business organisations like steel plants, heavy industries, etc. These cannot be run only with land, labour, capital and natural resources; highly capable managers are a must to design, direct and control various complex activities like marketing, selling, production, profit planning, industrial relations, etc.

Management and Market: The larger the market and more complicated the market structure, the greater is the intensity of use of managerial resources. For competitive pricing, packaging, distribution and advertising, highly competent management is required.

Capital Investment: The higher the capital investment in an enterprise, the greater the need for managerial talent, to ensure a profitable return on investments.

Innovation and Resources: Innovations, diversifications and modernisation of any kind often require heavy investment and call for high level managerial resources. The individual inventor is being replaced by large industrial research and control laboratories and research and development departments in all major industries.

Management and Productivity: 'Management is the principal factor determining the productivity if we assume that other factors of production are the same.

Studies have revealed that other things such as capital, modern machinery, technology and other factors being equal, sometimes achieve higher productivity which is often due to the efforts put in by talented managers and competent management.

Organisational Frictions: There are inherent frictions and personality clashes in most managerial organisations. Within most organisations there are professional jealousies, rivalries, conflicts of ideas, cliques, factions, alleged favouritism, etc., which decrease the efficiency of the organisation. Experienced managers know that "jockeying for positions" and "playing politics" consume a substantial portion of their energy. In making any vital decision one is apt to ask oneself, "how will it affect my position in the organisation". Such organisational frictions should be minimised. Frank and fearless views from managers should be welcomed rather than encouraging "yes sir" officers.

(ii) System of Authority

That management is a system of authority is evident from the fact that, for successful implementation of the policies, plans and objectives of the organisation, the management has to exercise its authority over its employees:

(i) Within management group

(ii) Over workers

Authority within groups: The most primitive system of management is sovereign rule by a single person or a single family without delegating authority to the middle management. It works only at the top and, when the top disappears, the organisation either collapses or necessitates rebuilding.

The modern theory of management lays emphasis on

"objectivity and self-control". Here the job of the top manager is to assist and develop managers under him by delegating authority and responsibility. The powers of top management are no doubt decentralised among various divisional managers but the ultimate policy decision, co-operation and control is normally left to the top boss.

Authority over Workers. While exercising control over workers, the management expects the following response from the workers:

- discipline
- loyalty to the management
- team work and collective efforts
- higher productivity and profits

Various theories or philosophies of management for exercising control over the workers have been put forward. Prominent among, these are:

(i) Dictatorial or authoritarian
(ii) Paternalistic
(iii) Constitutional
(iv) Democratic or participative.

Dictatorial or Authoritarian

According to this theory, the management should control the workers ruthlessly i.e., in a dictatorial way. It is felt that then alone will workers work more and be loyal. This philosophy, commonly found in private contractors, is primitive and is considered inadequate in a modern industrial atmosphere. Modern management researchers often stress that management should be inspiring and not driving; it should be firm but at the same time fair.

Paternalistic

Industrialisation of Japan is attributed to the paternalistic philosophy of its industrial management. According to this philosophy, the needs of the workers and their welfare are well taken care of by the management and in return the management expects that the workers would be loyal, disciplined and productive. Here the role of the manager is that of a benevolent autocrat.

Constitutional

In constitutional philosophy, while exercising control over workers, the management has to be aware of government legislations and pressures from various labour unions. Government forms' legislations to regulate conditions of employment as also to protect the growth of labour organisations, ensure proper working environments, welfare needs, etc. Yet workers/unions often challenge the authority of the management. In such cases, both the workers and the management are bound to settle their disputes within the frame-work of the prescribed rules. No side can take the law in its own hands and act in any manner it likes.

Democratic or Participative

The theory behind democratic or participative philosophy is, that free people respond best to an organisation when they can, participate in the process of decision-making on matters that directly, concern them. As per this system, workers should be encouraged, to participate in management decision-making or process and should shoulder equal responsibility. Representatives of workers or workers unions are inducted at various levels of decision-making, including up to the level of Board of Directors in some industrial undertakings/ organisations.

(iii) A Class or Elite

Management as a class is essentially a group of people, small in number, but aggressive in nature, who enjoy very high privileges and positions in society. These can be classified as:

Patrimonial Managers: Here members of the management group are members of the family which owns the enterprise or their chosen representatives.

Political Managers: This system exists where ownership, major policy-making positions and key administrative posts are held by persons on the basis of political affiliations and loyalties. It is generally practised or found in communist countries.

Professional Managers: Here the management positions are held by persons on the basis of their managerial and technical competence obtained by experience, qualifications or training rather than by family or political affiliations. The present trend is mostly towards engaging professional, talented and competent managers specially in large and technologically complex industries.

CLASSIFICATION ACCORDING TO FUNCTIONS

Katz and Kahn have given a classification, based on the functions performed, of an organisation. These are:

(1) Production or Economic Organisation

Such an organisation is concerned with "the creation of wealth, the manufacture of goods and the providing of services for the general public or the specific segments of it." Manufacturing organisations come under this category.

(2) Maintenance Organisation

This type of an organisation is "devoted to the socialisation of people for their roles in other organisations and in the larger society." Schools, social and cultural organisations come under this category.

(3) Adaptive Organisation

The object of such an organisation is to "create knowledge, develop and test theories and to some extent apply information to existing problems." Universities, research institutes, arts and science academies come under this category.

(4) Managerial or Political Organisation

Managerial or political organisations deal with the "adjudication, coordination and control of resources, people and subsystems." The State, labour unions and the professional bodies of doctors, lawyers, technicians, etc., are examples of this type of organisation.

The above differentiations are, however, not clear-cut. A single organisation may engage itself in more than one function. An economic organisation may take up the adaptive function also. Research divisions, for instance, form an important part of many manufacturing organisations. In supporting the above classifications, Katz and Kahn have considered major organisational characteristics as they interact with these major functions.

CLASSIFICATION ACCORDING TO SYSTEM

Organisations can be approached from a closed or open system perspective. Traditionally an organisation was considered sufficiently independent so that its formal structure and the relationships among its members could be established without reference to external situations. This is the closed system model view. The machine model or the bureaucratic form of organisation is identified with the close system. The open system model looks on an organisation not only from the viewpoint of its goals, objectives and its formal structure, but also from its response to the external environment and internal pressures. This refers to the contingency model which modern theorists advocate.

The bureaucratic or the closed system of organisation can be dimensionalised in the following ways:

(i) a division of labour based on functional specification;

(ii) a well-defined hierarchy of authority;

(iii) a system of rules covering the rights and duties of employees;

(iv) a system of procedures for dealing with work situation;

(v) impersonality of internal personal relations; and

(vi) promotion and selection of employees based on qualifications and competence.

The closed system developed as a reaction against the personal subjugation, nepotism and subjective judgment of administrators. It aimed at developing a rational structure of organisation, based on "tradition rather than cult of personality" and "technical competence" rather than whims. But when the rules, regulations and procedures become ends in themselves rather than becoming the means to achieve the ends, the organisations become rigid and inflexible.

The open system view recognises that the biological or social system is in a dynamic relationship with its environment and receives various inputs, transforms these inputs in some way and exports output.

Input → Transformation System → Output

The open system consists of a number of sub-systems. These are:

- Internal organisation (Organisational goals, values, etc.)
- Technical sub-system (Knowledge and techniques

required to transform inputs into output)

- Psychological sub-system (individual behaviour, motivation, status and role relationships, group dynamism, etc.)
- Structure (Organisation chart, job description, authority, communication, etc.)
- Managerial sub-systems (Developing strategies, plans, controls, etc.)
- Environmental sub-systems (Legal framework, government policy, economic and social environment, etc.).

The managerial decisions in the open system are contingent on the circumstances: Different organisations, with different tasks and different competitive environments, require different plans. The system, therefore, regards managers as a dynamic and life-giving force in the organisation.

Various factors such as the social, cultural or economic set-up of a country influence organisation or management of an enterprise. We, therefore, observe many instances of lack of uniformity in the pattern or philosophy of management. One has to choose an organisation that provides for cordial employer-employee relations, higher productivity, lower cost, security and welfare of workers, discipline, industrial safety, technological advancement, professional growth, etc.

CORPORATE OBJECTIVES AND POLICY FORMULATIONS

The objectives of management specify the goal towards which management aims, whereas policies provide guidelines which help attain that goal. The top management of successful enterprises defines the company objectives so that the management knows what the company stands for and the goals it has to achieve. A clear definition of the scope, responsibility and authority within which. the company has to operate is a must.

Based on the framework of corporate objectives, departmental policy manuals are drawn which like wise define, amplify and detail the departmental functions to help achieve the corporate objectives of the company. Drawing up of or laying down of corporate objectives appears simple, but is a very difficult, task in actual practice. These require long deliberations at top management level to clear the concepts before these could be defined and projected.

We shall discuss in detail the objectives as laid down by one of the Government of India undertakings to form an idea as to how that undertaking proposes to conduct its business. The said company operates large integrated steel plants in the country and being a government undertaking, is morally bound to the national goal of ensuring rapid economic growth through efficient production and supply of high quality iron, steel and allied products at reasonable rates.

The objectives of the company stem from the following major premises:

- As a public sector undertaking accountable to the people of India, the company will strive to maintain a sense of national interest in discharging its responsibilities and will constantly seek to deserve and enjoy the highest measure of public trust and esteem.
- In conducting its business with honesty and integrity, the company will also endeavour to function as a profitable enterprise striving towards the achievement of a self-reliant and self-generating economy.
- The company will operate in the highly specialised fields of iron and steel manufacture, and pioneer in

new fields of applied science through the pooling of the best scientific and engineering talent in an environment which will facilitate the proper utilisation of their knowledge, interest and skill.

- The operations of the company will be led by a management group which will enjoy the respect of the whole organisation for its ability, integrity, fairness and human approach to problems.
- As a high rate of economic growth sustained over a long period is the essential prerequisite for achieving a rising standard of living for the people, within the limits of resources it can generate, the company will seek to increase investment in basic production capacities and economic and social overheads so as to yield benefits now and in the future.
- The company will ensure good corporate health by adopting sound management practices, including the establishment and maintenance of a dynamic organisational structure suited to meet present and future company needs; long-range planning; product diversification; strong financial control and comprehensive research, development, engineering and consultancy services.

OBJECTIVES

Towards the People in India

— As an autonomous body, the company will be accountable to the people of India through Parliament and the government, for running a highly competent, business-minded, technically-oriented enterprise, engaging in manufacture, research and development to meet the needs of the country as well as world markets for iron, steel and allied products.

- The company will endeavour to earn a fair return on the investment, maximise production, institute adequate cost control, so managed as to inspire confidence and a sense of pride in the minds of the people.

Towards Employees

The company will seek to be a model employer by:

- attracting competent personnel with growth potential and by developing their maximum capabilities in a working environment through the provision of opportunities for advancement and incentives;
- developing and sustaining a favourable employee attitude and obtaining maximum contribution of employees through stable employment; adequate wages commensurate with the company's capacity to pay; good and safe working conditions and job satisfaction;
- establishing a system for redressal of employees' grievances in the shortest possible time and at the lowest possible step;
- providing training facilities and other opportunities for self-development in their current jobs and for further advancement;
- fostering fellowship and a sense of belonging to the company through closer association of employees with management by way of participation in various joint bodies and through this machinery inculcating in them respect for their occupation and for the tools of production;
- by dealing fairly with recognised representatives of workers, and encouraging in them healthy trade union practices.

Towards Customers

The company will serve its customers by:.

- providing prompt, courteous, dependable and competitive services;
- selling products of the right quality at prices determined in the best interests of the nation; and,
- establishing confidence in the customers that it will supply the required products and services backed by modern production and research facilities manned by the most competent men available.

Towards Suppliers

The company recognises the important role of its suppliers in providing various materials and services in its operations by:

- ensuring prompt dealings based on integrity, impartiality and courtesy, making available to them the benefits of research, skills and information in order to promote indigenous growth, reduce drain on foreign exchange and improve the quality of indigenous products and services.

Towards the Community

The company accepts its social obligations to the community in which it operates by:

- promoting the concept of national integration in its broadest sense, through providing community services, developing and assisting democratic institutions and generally ensuring that the company as a whole and its employees act on the ideals of social justice without discrimination;
- providing know-how and assistance, and encouraging talent and growth among members of the community through the establishment of cooperative institutions.

The company endeavours to be one of the most enlightened, progressive and efficient producers of iron and steel and allied products in India and abroad, by making the most effective use of capital, personnel and management skills.

Whereas it is important to set the goals in as detailed and specific a manner as possible, it is wrong to assume that corporate objectives will be all inclusive and do the job alone. The respective departments of the company have to have their own policy manuals further amplifying the action to be taken by them to help achieve the overall objectives.

For example, if the top management declares in its corporate objectives that, wherever practicable, the deliveries of the items have to be made on the stipulated dates and that no extension of dates would generally be granted. The production planning and control department, in that case, has to study each order in detail and give a delivery schedule only after a very careful study of the various factors involved. The production planning and control department will then be obliged to set up a system of follow-up and corrective action to meet this requirement. The system is to be so designed and controlled for reliability as to see that this objective is honoured.

Large companies often employ systems and procedures managers who help the departmental heads in preparing policy manuals for their departments. Depending on the circumstances, such as political changes; change of government/board of directors controlling the company; declaration of war, declaration of national emergency; etc., the objectives of a company may undergo changes or show signs of changes or drifts. The top executives should keep themselves up-to-date in this respect but use their discretion and judgment in communicating a part or the whole of this change down the line to specified positions in the hierarchy.

MANAGEMENT BY OBJECTIVES

While speaking of objectives, it may be useful to know about a recent style in management known as MBO or management by objectives. It is a dynamic system which seeks to integrate the needs of the enterprise along with the growth of their managers. It is a demanding and rewarding style of management.

Peter F. Drucker in his book *Practice of Management* has described in a very lucid manner as to:

- what the needs of *team-spirit* are
- why *objectives* are a must
- what the forces *of misdirection* are
- how these can be *coordinated*
- when management by *drive* develops
- who should set *objectives.*

and what the advantages of Management by Objectives (MBO) are.

Team Spirit

Business enterprises must build a team and for this efforts must be put in the same direction; contributions must fit together to produce a worthwhile team—without cracks or without friction, without unnecessary duplication of efforts. Business performance, therefore, requires that each job be directed towards the objective of the whole business. The collective spirit is the essence that matters.

Misdirection

The managers must know and understand what business goals demand of them in terms of performance, and their superiors must know what contributions to demand and expect of them. They must be judged on that scale. Managers are not automatically directed towards a common goal. The directions are to come from the top and are to be carefully explained to the hierarchy below in a simple and understandable manner. Unless a man knows precisely his goals, his efforts may be misdirected and may lead to infructuous activity.

There are generally three powerful forces of misdirection:

- Specialised work of most managers
- Hierarchical structure of management
- Difference in vision and work

The functional managers' legitimate desire for workmanship (unless counter-balanced) causes a centrifugal force which tears the enterprise apart and converts it into a loose confederation of functional empires, each concerned only with its own craft, each jealously guarding its own secrets, each bent on enlarging its own domain rather than on building the business.

The future technologies will need both the drive for excellence in workmanship and the consistent direction of managers at all levels towards common goals.

The hierarchical system of dictatorial management often creates speculations. What the boss does and says, his most casual remarks, his habits, even his mannerisms, tend to appear to his subordinates as calculated, planned and meaningful. This happens where the hierarchy believes in and suffers from the 'Yes Sir' complex and despises logic or logistics of the situation.

Drive

Drive without a proper goal or guidance misleads the management. During a misdirected "economy drive", for instance—a few people may be fired. But this hardly offers any solution. Similarly for unplanned and abrupt "inventory cut drive", there may be four weeks of cost cutting, followed by four months of production and human relations problems.

Management by *drive* or *crisis* is an admission of incompetence. It is a sign that management does not know how to plan. Above all, it is a sign that company does not know what to expect of its managers.

Each manager should develop and set objectives of his unit himself. Higher management must, of course, reserve the power to approve or disapprove these objectives. The objectives of a district sales manager, for example, should be defined by the contribution he and his district sales force make towards the sales department.

Some advocate that each subordinate should write to his senior about the objectives he feels are expected of him and the objectives of his superior. Further, he should list his own responsibilities and the difficulties he may envisage. His expectations and the help he expects from his superiors for fulfilling his tasks should also be outlined.

Each manager from the "big boss" down to the production foreman or the chief clerk needs clearly spelled out objectives. These objectives should specify:

- the performance he and his unit are supposed to make;
- the contribution he and his unit are expected to make to help other units obtain their objectives.
- the contribution the manager expects from other units towards the attainment of his objectives;

Right from the start the emphasis should be on *team work* and *team spirit* and *team result*. It is the proper synchronisation and tuning of collective efforts that produce the results.

Coordination

The solution to this problem requires a structure of management which focuses both the manager's and his boss's eyes on what they job is rather than what the *boss* demands.

Each level of management sees the same elephant—the business—from a different angle of vision. The production foreman sees only the immediate production problems. The quality foreman is interested only in his quality specifications. The top management only tends to see the enterprise as a whole. An effective management must direct the vision, and coordinate the efforts of all managers towards a common goal.

Advantages of M.B.O.

Some of the specific advantages of Management by Objectives (MBO) are:

1. It makes possible for a manager to control his own performance. Self-control means stronger motivation—a desire to do the best rather than just enough to get by. It means higher performance goals and broader vision.
2. It enables us to substitute management by self-control for management by domination.
3. It enables complete rethinking on oar use of reports, procedures and forms. Procedures should not be a substitute for judgment. They should be at best regarded as tools and an aid to decision-making.
4. MBO rests on the concept of human action, human behaviour and human motivation.

Story of Ford and MBO

In the early twenties Ford's share market of the automobile had climbed to over 60 per cent. Fifteen years later it went down by *20* per cent. Ford's only son died during World War II. Survival of the company seemed impossible. There was talk either to nationalise it to give loans to Studebaker Company, the fourth largest automobile producer of the US, to buy up Ford Motors which was less than one-sixth of the size of the Ford.

What was the cause? The fundamental mistake of Henry Ford was that he made a systematic, deliberate and conscious attempt to run the billion dollar business without managers. The secret police that spied on all Ford executives served to inform Henry Ford of any attempt on the part of any of his executives to make a decision. When they seemed to acquire managerial authority or responsibility of their own, their services were generally dispensed with.

Henry Ford wanted only technicians and reserved management to himself as the owner. He did not like sharing either ownership or management with others. It was thus the absence of management which was responsible for the fall of Ford Motors.

Later, it was Henry Ford II (the grandson of Ford) who reversed the old policies. He appointed Earnest B. Bruch as Vice-President of the Company and gave him full operating authority. This concept was observed by setting up different managerial cadres with defined objectives throughout the organisation.

Management came to be governed by management by objectives. Whereas Ford executives under the old regime were never told anything, the new Henry regime tried to provide every manager with the information he needed to do his job. The company was decentralised into various operating autonomous divisions, each, with its own complete management. Ford II took most of these ideas from his competitors (General Motors) and thus saved Ford Motors from closure.

When a system of Management by objectives is operating in an enterprise there is a continuous process of:

(a) Reviewing critically and re-specifying the enterprise's *strategic and tactical plans.*

(b) Specifying the *key results and performance standards* which each manager must achieve so as to fulfil the objectives of the enterprise and gain his share from it.

(c) Inspiring and driving each manager to carry out *a job improvement plan* which makes a measurable and realistic contribution to the units and company's plan for better performance.

(d) Providing and maintaining conditions in which it is possible to achieve the key results and improvement plans like an *organisation structure* which gives a manager maximum freedom and flexibility in decision-making and execution.

(e) Installing an effective *management information system* which gives *timely* information in required *frequency* and in an *understandable* manner for quick decision and corrective action.

(f) Holding systematic *performance reviews* to critically measure the progress achieved against norms/targets and locating potential for leadership to deliver the goods.

(g) Developing managers through management training and development programmes, and better motivation by effective selection, salary and promotion plans. A manager must be able to pinpoint unimportant deviations indicating need for corrective action.

We may conclude that MBO is a system of business-management whereby the enterprise tries to utilise and develop to the fullest extent its most precious resource—managers—to achieve its goals. It integrates the company's objectives for profit and growth with the personal goals and satisfaction of its managers. It is an established fact now that the key to real success in business depends on effective use of its human resources, their talent, initiative, dynamism and ability to deliver the goods.

REFERENCES

1. Maslow, A.H. (1954), *Motivation and Personality.* New York, Harper & Row Publishers.
2. Vroom, Victor H. (1978), *Work and Motivation.* Wiley Eastern Ltd., p. 197.

4

CONCEPTS OF HUMAN RESOURCE PLANNING

"Enthusiasts without capaicty are the really dangerous people."

—*John Morley*

"Success or failure in business is caused more by mental attitudes than by mental capacities."

—*Walter Dill Scott*

Recognition of 'Human Capital' or 'Human Resource' is rather a new phenomenon in arena of Development. Earlier in the process of production it was termed as 'Labour.' The early development planners over-emphasised the role of physical capital in economic growth. However the development literature of the 1950s and 1960s paid ample attention to the role of human beings as human capital, and by 1970s it recognised the development of human resources as the most crucial objective.

Human Resource Development, has taken centre stage in the development debate. This is not one day too early, since the human condition and what can be done to improve it are close to the objectives of development than are the means and material requisites which have long been the preoccupation of economic development planners and policy-makers.

Human resources development (HRD) is the process of increasing the knowledge, the skills, and the capacities of all the people in the society. In economic terms, it could be described as the accumulation of human capital and its effective investment in the development of an economy. In political terms, human resource development prepares people for adult participation in political processes. From the social and cultural points of view, the development of human resources helps people lead fuller and affluent lives.

The concept of HRD has two facets—first, dealing with human resource development and second, with regard to its utilisation. There are several inputs which are required for the development and utilisation of human resources. For example, nutrition, drinking water, health, education, training, sports, culture, housing and communication etc. may be considered as critical for a proper development of these resources. Keeping in view the long gestation period that is required before the investment in human resources can start bearing fruit, it is necessary to have a continued commitment for the purpose.

Human resources are developed in many ways *i.e.*, through formal-education, on-the-job training, self development, improvement of health and nutrition. HRD related activities seek to design, redesign and continuously upgrade the potential of human resources so that the latter continues to contribute to the process of development in a productive manner. This has to be so irrespective of the stage of economic growth and any particular phase through which the economy may be passing. It requires a detailed exercise in which the specificities of the society are especially taken note of. Thus planning and management of human resources becomes a perennial exercise.

Many common supportive and trade-off linkages are there among the different components which go into the making of human resources. Hence it requires an integrated approach and one has to take a holistic view of the conditions under which human resources are suppored to be developing. More importantly, it is also clear that the combinations of these inputs may vary from period to period or from one situation to another.

Integrated Human Resources Development

Basically, 'Integrated human resources development' is a broad concept covering a full range of social and economic development processes. It is an approach to overall development that places the well-being of the people first and regards human beings as both agents as well as beneficiaries of all development efforts. The concern in integrated human resources development is no just on improving purely work and productivity-related human capabilities such as employment and manpower development but all aspects that are vital to the improvement of the welfare of the people and their active participation in the development process. It recognises that human resources development is influenced by, as well as effects, a whole array of social, economic and cultural variables, and that it can be best served by a board range of 'interventions' or 'strategies'. The objectives of integrated human resources development go beyond adoption of a larger and more diverse set of social interventions. It seeks to develop human resources in a concerted and coherent manner by incorporating all aspects and phases of socio-economic development into human resources development planning.

In an integrated human resources development approach, strategies will not just tend to be demand-oriented. The creation of human resources must be coordinated with their effective utilisation. Instead of just regulating the supply of labour through population controls, integrated human resources development policies seek to remove all obstacles and provide opportunities to ensure a conducive environment for the full and productive utilisation of human resources. Investments in physical and human infrastructure are also to be coordinated. The whole essence is to maximise returns to development efforts and optimise distribution of its benefits. However, although the human resources development approach advocates an inter-agency holistic approach, it also recognises that, in certain countries budgetary and manpower constraints, dictate a more focused approach limited to a selected number of major issues and target groups instead of a comprehensive approach. For comprehensive development planning, human resources variables must be considered in their broad perspective, and this can only be achieved through strong coordination in human resources development policy-making, planning and programming.

Early Reservations

The classical economists had all through recognised the role of human resources in the development of production capabilities as well as in sustaining the broader social structure. But notwithstanding this, they, shunned away from treating human beings as means of production. The main school of economic thought, as represented by Adam Smith, J.S. Mill and Alfred Marshall held on to this position, even while acknowledging the productive role of human resources.

Human Beings as Capital

During the late nineteenth and first half of twentieth century, when the requirement for the workers in the developed countries, particularly in the United States of America was at its peak, the need for mass education to equip people with the requisite traits was felt. The emergence of opinion in favour of mass education and pervasive growth of "educational industry" in United States of America during this period was in a way a reflection of the scale at which industrial development required trained human resources.

The process continued during the early period of the twentieth century. It can be said that it came to its full, around the World War II. It is in this phase of industrial growth the linkages between education and employment, reached its climax. Consequently in the fifties, educational sector got recognised as a critical component of the growth process. The realisation led to the discovery of "human factor" and development analysis heralded the human capital revolution. Schultz, Harbison, Meyers and Becker led the parade which opened up several new areas of economic analysis including health, welfare, poverty and home economics.

Manpower

Generally speaking, Manpower is a macro-concept referring to an aggregate of categories of skilled personnel; distinct and separate categories of manpower are identifiable on the basis of the level and type of their skills; and these skills are generated by means of education and training, both within the formal education system and outside.

In current popular usage, the terms manpower", "labour", "labour force", "work force" and "human resources" are all being employed as though they are conceptually identical or as mere variants in expression; however, no harm could possibly be done by indiscriminate use of these terms to theory and analysis, provided their specific, distinct and separate meaning are identified and kept in mind constantly.

Sometimes the word manpower is equivalent to the term labour when labour is understood to be a factor of production in the basic framework of analysis used by economists. In this very broad sense manpower can also be understood to mean generically "personnel" or "employees". Actually these usages of the term are virtually identical; the differences are less in substance than in point of view, one being that of the labour economist and the other that of the personnel student or practitioner.

Viewed at in still another manner, manpower can mean the total quantitative and qualitative human assets or people in a society. In this sense we are literally interpreting the word to mean the power of man, both in terms of the size of the population and the talents and educational levels in that population. Population can be said to determine the quantity, and education combined with experience, the quality, of manpower. During World War II, when there was a War Manpower Commission, manpower seemed to have the latter connotations.

It is noteworthy here that it is conceptually invalid to equate "labour" with "Manpower". Similarly the term "human resources" is also not identical with "Manpower" since it is more generic including both skilled and unskilled categories of workers. Further manpower is also different from the term "labour force" used in surveys of employment and unemployment. Because labour force constitutes "workers + unemployed". Finally the term "Working Force" denotes but a component of labour force that is engaged in-gainful activity.

Manpower thus denotes definite and specific categories which are in theory : (1) non-homogeneous and are therefore, (2) non- substitutable. To take a typical example: A doctor (from the category of medical manpower) is non-substitutable from an engineer (from the category of technical manpower). However, within each category it is possible to substitute one unit for another, provided the second has skills indentical with those of the first.

Manpower Planning

Essentially, planning is a process of thinking ahead, a method for anticipating difficulties and seeking, through reasoned action based upon fore-knowledge, to guide the course of events toward desired goals. By this means, planning approaches the future with the aid of systematic analysis in order to minimise, surprise and uncertainty and to eliminate mistakes and waste.

Manpower planning in economic terms applies the processes of planning in general to the preparation and employment of people for productive purposes. Manpower planning may thus be viewed as a tool of manpower policy. At national level, manpower planning aims to enlarge job opportunities and improve training and employment decisions through the power of informed personnel choice and calculated adjustment to rapidly changing demand. By means of more intelligent training and career decisions and greater adaptability of the nation's labour force, manpower planning may enhance satisfaction in a job, raise the quality and utilisation of manpower, reduce the cost of job search and industry staffing, and, thereby, increase the output of a nation.

First, manpower planning may be viewed in the very narrow sense of replacement planning as that term is normally used in the conduct of industrial relations activities in organisations. From this standpoint, manpower planning encompasses the analysis of labour turnover, thinking through personnel recruitment policies, identifying approaches to the planning of careers for employees, developing models for planning recruitment and the promotion of employees and analysing the relationship between pay policies and recruitment.

Secondly, manpower planning is to consider it tantamount to personnel planning, that is, the planning carried out by the staff personnel department as opposed to the administrative work. Personnel planning ranges over all activities of the department, includes recruitment, selection, placement, training, education wage and salary administration, safety, labour relations, and like. This definition is obviously considerably broader than viewing manpower planning as programming the organisational staffing.

Thirdly, manpower planning applies to manpower and employment policy at the level of the economy. In this framework "manpower" is regarded as the quantitative and qualitative measurement of a nation's labour force, and "planning" is regarded as establishing objectives and programmes to develop human resources in line with various other goals. Very often the focus in this type of manpower planning is primarily on highly trained manpower and its role in the development of an underdeveloped country. Or, conversely, it may be on the most poorly educated manpower in an urban-industrial society and what is required (in terms of education, training, health improvement, and the like) to bring these human resources into the mainstream of society. This point of view typically becomes involved with demography, the population composition in terms of educational levels, age and sex ratios, the skill mix, and present and future gross national product.

Finally, manpower planning is the process by which an organisation ensures that it has the right number of people and the right kind of people, at the right places, at the right time doing for which they are economically most useful. It is therefore, a two-phased process, by which we anticipate the future through manpower projections and then develop and implement manpower action plans and programmes to accommodate the projection implications.

Human Resource

Similar to the concept of manpower, the concept of human resources has many different meanings, stripped of subtleties, both manpower and human resources refer to and mean people. Human resources could be equated with "labour" in the sense of a factor of production, or simply population. Human resources may also be viewed as a kind of natural resource or a people resource just as we have mineral and forest resources.

Development

One is by formal education, beginning with primary or

first-level education, continuing through various forms of secondary education, and then culminating in higher education, including colleges, universities, and technical institutes. Second, human resources are developed on-the-job through systematic or informal training programmes in employing institutions; in adult education programmes; and through membership in various political, social, religious, and other groups. A third way is through self-development, as persons seek to acquire greater knowledge, skills, or capacities through preparation on their own initiative, such as taking formal correspondence courses, reading, or learning from others in informal contacts. Motivation for self-development varies from society to society. It is directly related to the social values in a culture, to incentives for training and entering one occupation rather than another, and to incentives for learning new skills. Planning for development of human resources is very essential and hence the need for *human resource planning (HRP).* At the terms Manpower Planning and human resource planning are used to refer to planning for the development of people they can be used interchangeably

Manpower Planning

All organisations plan to some extent, even though the plans may consist of no more than a few general ideas carried around in the heads of top managers and based on an informal forecast derived from past, experience, known facts, common sense, and a few hunches. Planning of this type needs no explanation because, it is tantamount to rational thinking. Our interest is in formal planning in which definite techniques and procedures are used and written plans are produced. Formal planning systems as viewed in the perspective of managing large-scale organisations are a relatively new arrival on the mangerial scene. Overall "master planning" or "corporate planning" was given impetus principally by World War II when organisations engaged in war work realised that the end of hostilities would mean they could no longer sell a large proportion of their output to the government and they would have to find new customers, if not new products, if they hoped to stay in business. An incipient need for manpower planning was also evident at this time. After 1940, many organisations experienced manpower shortages as a conquence of production needs during the World War II period, which ran from late 1941 to almost the end of 1945, and the entry of millions of young men and women into the armed forces. This period was preceded by a long depression and marked the prewar defense mobilisation period. In the depression manpower problems were considered essentially employment problems because of the large number of unemployed persons. In the defense period prior to Pearl Harbor, and particularly after the entry of the United States into the war, manpower shortages developed in various industries.

The ideas of "postwar planning", gradually spread from organisations concerned mainly with war production to companies producing entirely for civilian markets because it was evident that peace and the end of wartime shortages would change their environment drastically. As a result, corporate planning was added to the list of important managerial functions for many organisations. Even without this push it is likely that formal corporate planning would have developed rapidly at this time, primarily as a consequence of industrial growth, technological change, and social trends. Another cause of postwar planning was the increasing technical complexity of many products as well as their faster obsolescence.

This meant that, before a company would go ahead with a product requiring expensive, research and development, it wanted some assurance through planning and forecasting that sales would be large enough and continue over a long enough period of time to make the investment worthwhile.

In turn, this led to profit planning in which objective were set and plans were made to insure that all parts of the organisation were geared toward the accomplishment of those objectives by means of specific plans. Automation further increased the need for long-range planning.

Turning from industrial interest in long-range or postwar planning and manpower planning, it should be noted that there has been an emerging interest for many years in manpower and human resources on the part of educational, governmental, military, and other organisations.

Since the end of World War II, the development of active manpower policies in both industrial and developing countries has created a demand for advanced information about manpower changes. In the underdeveloped countries, which have an over-supply of unskilled labour shortages of high trained and educated manpower, emphasis has been on the supply of high and middle-level manpower.

Besides this, many people have been concerned whether educational requirements are outstripping educational attainment. Still others have asked questions whether the skills that are being supplied are those which are really in demand now and will continue to be in the future. This fear and fascination with employment and manpower problems has created a renewed interest in predicting the future as well as caused considerable frustration with some of the existing indicators of what the state of manpower will be at that time.

The effect of this interest in the future has been to tax the energies and intellectual limits of specialists in manpower planning and to have led those who wish information on manpower planning to make demands on manpower specialists which are unrealistic given the existing state of knowledge. Manpower planning to be viewed in the context of a society and its prevailing cultural values. In this way, one can obtain an appreciation of the direction which manpower planning has taken in the economy and understand the implications of this direction for industrial organisations. In this way, one shall obtain 'some insight into why manpower planning has become a relatively new activity in industrial relations and why its importance will undoubtedly grow in the future.

Manpower planning essentially makes projections of supply and demand of Manpower. These projections of the supply and demand for manpower may be utilised for a variety of purposes. These include (1) planning educational programmes and estimating what expansions in enrollment must be provided for in order to meet future needs for workers of all types, (2) evaluating the feasibility of launching new programmes requiring skilled personnel, (3) the vocational guidance of individuals, (4) developing manpower programmes and policies. Essentially, manpower projections are useful for two prime purposes: to alert the government and other organisations to emerging manpower problems; and to provide a basis for educational planning, counselling, and guidance.

The important thing for us to note is that the recognition of human resources as a factor of production, brackets it along with other artefacts, in which investment of capital can be undertaken. The hypothesis provided a rationale for changing the public policy in favour of more resources into all kinds of social services including education, training, health and nutrition. The ethos of the period dominated the development strategy of the sixties.

What do we know about transforming raw human resources into knowledgeable, skilled and trained manpower? Although it is possible to pose this question in a more comprehensive manner, we eschew the same here and focus on the problem as stated.

Traditionally, the manpower training question has always been looked at from the point of view of supply side. It is presumed that economic growth assumes a certain quantities of skilled personnel in the absence of which the process itself stands arrested. Hence manpower planners attempt to ensure a steady supply of trained personnel with requisite qualifications to meet the growing demand.

Whereas there is no disagreement upto this point, one has to pinpoint the stage of readiness upto which education prepares a person and at what stage his on-the-job induction training begins. It is well known that this kind of approach assumes a strict one-to-one correspondence between educational process and job market It assumes a certain rigid view of production technology.

If there is a strict relationship between education and matching of graduates to the job slot, then the main things which one needs to do are:

(a) estimate demand for manpower in terms of different skills knowledge,

(b) link the required skills /knowledge with certain levels of educational programmes, and

(c) invest inputs in the educational sector, both, human as well as material to produce the stream, of graduates.

It is obvious that the assumption about production technologies and matching of graduates with jobs is quite flexible in the latter version. To. that extent planning of manpower is different in the two formulations. In the former it is strictly technologically determined while in the latter, it is determined by market forces with varying degree of public policy.

Remarkably the use of information in these two types of situation and the nature of their organisation is quite different from each other. The former takes off on the hardware governed by engineering notion of a workplace wherein a worker with certain profile and skills fits into the system as a counterpart to the machine. In the latter there is greater fuzziness. The organisation of production and requisite skills, are identified and transacted by the market relation. What skills are going to be in demand and are going to be supplied by educational institutions is governed by commercialisations of yield and profitability. Consequently in this interpretation there is a room for skill substitution. There is also greater role of information and organisation of production in this case. It is not the production hardware, but organisational relations of production systems, which determine the manpower generation and depolyment decisions.

Education and Training

One of the major outcome of this pressure is that the basic relationship between education and manpower is undergoing vital change. Education is no more being looked as an institution in which the potential 'factory mates' are being given rudiments of essential knowledge with a view to make them better workers. It is also not a place where only generic education is being provided and that the pupils are being certified with regard to their class, performance ability and other attributes.

It see that the certification function of education is now going to undergo a decline with diminishing role of public sector and public policy of employment and recruitment. The emphasis today is to increase and tap the creative aspect of human intelligence. Manpower has to do what machines cannot do as of now. It is the nature of information that is determining the pattern of education, manpower training and generation of modern skilled workers. The uncertainties about the production systems are not today in the realm of either their hardware or about the material to be used for the production, but about their interlinkages with the infrastructure, with transportation system, with communications, and in brief with their social environment in which these industries are going to be located.

HRD is no more simply another form of capital investment. Human resources are now emerging as an end in itself. The communication revolution, the shrinking size of the globe, the rapidly changing society, the threat of nuclear holocaust and the research for peace paradigm are all manifestations of a common underlying spirit—the spirit of homo sapiens.

Situation in Developing Countries

The succinctly described different phases of human resources are significant in describing the varying emphasis that the subject has undergone over the years. Needless to say that this was a stylised description in which several complications have been simplified. The way problem of human resources surface in the developing countries is even more complicated.

In the developing countries the technologies of the different vintages have to co-exist simultaneously and consequently the obtained profile of an economy and the society is highly stratified and segmented. Each layer has its own peculiar characteristics. Consequently, the development of the human resources has to be undertaken in an open-ended pluralistic manner with all kinds of positive discrimination policies for different groups. The result is that the programmes tend to be general and thc investment gets stretched to cover all types of diverse claims. This leads to under-investment, inefficiency, and interventions in the decision-making. It is in this type of setting that the problematique of HRD needs to be viewed for it to be relevant for the developing societies.

Arguing from apriori position it would seem that two opposite types of policy measures are required for tackling the problems that are being faced by these late developing countries. Firstly, they need to resort to modern technology for being able to provide services to a large number of people at low per unit cost. Secondly, they need to invest in the hi-tech areas to build bridgeheads which could facilitate the monitoring and indigenisation of the new knowledge and information. In other words, they need programmes of human resource which have the maximum impact on their population in terms of sheer coverage, and on top of it, with the help of high level manpower they need to be able to break new grounds in the realm of hi-tech. These two basic approaches span the policy options and contain within it the choice matrix relevant for the developing countries like India.

India an Scenario

Due to sectoral investment planning, the different components of HRD have had disjoined isolated approach in India. Consequently different members of the populace were identified as target group for different programmes. No coordinated planning for human resource development has been taken up. More importantly even where coordinated planning efforts were attempted their implementation could not be carried out in unison with other activities. No well-knit system exists at present to ensure coordination and integration of human resources development programmes in India. The responsibility for the implementation of human resources development is shared between the central and state governments, because planning for a country of India's size and diversity is not so easily organised, supervised and controlled by the centre. As the primary implementing agencies in human resources development, the state governments determine their own policies and also draw up their five year and annual plans of development. The central government, however, influences state policies, by initiating national level programmes in crucial areas, by developing and ensuring national standards, and providing substantial financial assistance to the states.

Planning Commission

The Planning Commission, headed by the Prime Minister, is responsible for scrutinizing the five year and annual plans of the states and the central government and matching them with the available resources and national priorities. Its main functions involve advice and coordination rather than implementation. Since it has the responsibility of developing perspective long-term plans as well as mid-term plans and annual plans, and undertakes evaluation, the Planning Commission is in a unique position to ensure the development of human resources and to monitor their implementation. It already contains the mechanism for coordination of many of the components of human resources development, particularly those relating to the social sector and quality of life, as it has a full-time commissioner in charge of human resources development, looking after health, social welfare, education, culture, women and child development, youth services and sports. The commissioner closely cooperates with other commissioners responsible for science and technology, employment, agriculture, rural development, and other related sectors. In a sense therefore, the Planning Commission has become a coordinating agency for human resources development in India.

Notably, Its coordination, however, is confined to policy and planning aspects. The executive responsibility for human resources development at the national level is shared by the Ministry of Human Resources Development; with other ministries such as the Ministry of Labour, which is responsible for technical training: of workers, the Department of Health which is responsible for the provision of health services, the Department of Science and Technology and various other institutes. Since the assigned role of the Ministry of Human Resources Development only addresses quality of life concern, programmes relating to health, employment and science and technology are outside its purview.

The Ministry of Human Resources Development comprises the Departments of Education, Culture, Youth Services and Sports, and Women and Child Development. The cabinet-level Minister of Human Resources Development is assisted by two State Ministers, one in charge of Education and Culture and another in charge of Youth Services and Sports, and Women and Child Development.

Institute of Applied Manpower Research

Established by the government in 1962 as an autonomous organisation, the institute functions under the aegis of the Planning Commission. It seeks to broaden awareness of manpower planning and manpower development issues, among like-minded institutions, central and state government departments, and public sector programmes through training, research, seminars, and conferences.

The Institute has established formal linkages with central ministries, state governments, public and private sector organisations, professional bodies, and academic and research institutions, through its Executive Council and Standing Committees on Research Programmes. Affiliated organisations participate in formulating the policies and programmes of the Institute. On occasions, they have also collaborated with the institute and aided its research on manpower and employment planning. The Institute's structure and linkages enable it to play an important role in developing a progressive philosophy among those formulating and implementing human resources development policies.

In summary, while it can be observed that there is no

single agency responsible for all human resources development coordination, a strong lead has been taken in this regard by the Ministry of Human Resources Development and the Institute of Applied Manpower Research, which have sought to establish linkages with other departments and agencies concerned with human resources development.

Several inter-ministerial committees function at various levels in India. A good example is the frequent and dose coordination between the Department of Health and the Department of Women and Child Welfare under the Integrated Child Development Scheme. The "technology mission" approach adopted for literacy programmes also provides for several coordinating committees among the departments themselves. Similar arrangements exist at the state-level in a number of states, wherein Secretaries have been placed in charge of human resources development.

A STRATEGY FOR FUTURE

In principle, human development is a comprehensive approach. In addition to the standard growth rates per capita, recognition is given to other measurable components like longevity and literacy and factors not easy to measure like human freedom and cultural attainments.

The first thing that strikes one about human development is that it is as comprehensive and composite a concept as development itself. It embraces social development as in the field of education and health. It calls for the participation of all sections of the population in the development process. It can be promoted best in an environment of human freedom and exercise of democratic, rights. It requires for itself a flourishing and sound framework for social justice and equality of opportunity; It recognises importance of our cultural roots, deriving inspiration from it, without getting trapped by the outdated modes and customs, and constantly keeping in mind the need to modernise it also calls for access to resources for leading a decent life diversifying ones choices.

Attention has now been focused increasingly on human development and its relationship with human freedoms—democracy and human rights.

It is important to note that the exercise of human freedoms by itself must construe expression of human development. They are pre-conditions for it, not the outcome of it, as the democratic process ensures suitable conditions for human development.

Now coming to the role of market forces in ensuring human development. Here there is a danger of exaggerating the role of market forces. There is no doubt that you cannot have human freedom unless you are very strong and not bound by want and deprivation. But free market forces themselves do not achieve this task. In the developed countries we have social welfare and security provisions, a hallmark of human development. The social welfare system has today become part and parcel of the socio-economic life of these countries.

In developing countries, we lack a comprehensive social security net, for want of resources, for want of a system of management; and, therefore, governments have to play a very important role to fill the gap. This function is exercised mainly in the form of organising activities directed at providing employment to those who are unable to find gainful work for want of skills and access to resources.

Massive resources are requiredin the human development areas. Human development is such a gigantic task that an effort has to be made to encourage the mobilisation of the resources of the developing countries, mainly by themselves. Second, unless they are themselves to be incharge of human development activities, the results are not going to be satisfactory. Human development is something which can hardly be brought about by providing expertise or by just making some equipment available.

The United Nations System concentrated on providing support with an emphasis on human development, in the earlier part of the technical assistance programme. Then, in the early 1950s and 60s the concentration was on economic growth. This had an effect on the UN's own priorities and very soon the emphasis shifted to pre-investment activities.

Sustainable Development

In population rich but land-hungry countries like India, China and Bangladesh, enduring food security will depend greatly on strategies to enhance crop yields. At the same time, the onward march of the green revolution will have to be on the basis of 'green' or environmental friendly technologies. If productivity-enhancing technologies do not spread to more areas and farming systems, the poverty of small farm families will persist, since they will have very little marketable surplus and thus will not be able to profit from the remunerative output-pricing policies of governments.

A major aim of the strategy described as Low Input Sustainable Agriculture (LISA) by the US Department of Agriculture is to ensure the long-term sustainability of current production levels in USA. However, while defending the status quo in yield may be the priority task in industrialised nations, raising average yields is the urgent need in developing countries. India already has over 47 per cent of its land area under agriculture. Every fourth farmer in the world is an Indian farmer. Less than 4 per cent of the arable land of the country is under pastures and grazing lands, although India has over 20 per cent of the world's farm animal population. Unless rice yields are doubled within the next 20 years, it will be difficult to manage the national food security system without food imports. The same situation prevails in wheat, sorghum, pulses, oilseeds, and other food crops. So the pathways for sustainable agriculture in India will have to be based on substantial advances in productivity and not just on the maintenance of current yields and production levels.

On the one hand, several of the components associated with traditional green revolution or land-saving technologies, particularly those involving the use of high doses of mineral fertilizers, chemical pesticides and heavy farm machinery, have negative ecological reprecussions. On the other hand, a continuous growth in terrestrial and aquatic productivity is a must in countries where agriculture holds the key not only to food security but to the livelihood security of rural families.

Sustainable agriculture has several dimensions — social, cultural and economic, besides ecological. This task is made complex in large countries like India not only by the numbers involved, but by the pressures of competing needs. Unless there is equity in sharing the benefits cooperation will not be easily forthcoming. This is true both within and among nations. We, therefore, need a new paradigm of agricultural research and development for enduring global and national food security, consisting of three interacting components—ecological sustainability, equity-based economic efficiency, and convergence and synergy among the efforts of the government, non-government and corporate sectors.

Successful genetic engineering needs access to a wide range of genetic resources of crops and animals.

The task of achieving sustainable advances in biological productivity is a formidable one. The progress made so far through changes in plant architecture and physiological responses is largely due to a higher allocation of the total biomass to the part of economic value. Further progress will depend on our ability to improve total biomas production per unit of land and water. This is where the tools of molecular biology have added to our research capability. The biological technologies essential to derive the necessary gene combinations through recombinant-DNA experiments are largely being perfected in the private sector in industrialised and developing nations.

REFERENCES

1. *Inter-organisational Coordination for Human Resources Development Policy Making, Planning and Programming,* UN-UNDP, New Year, 1991, pp. 5-7.
2. Wendall French, *The Personnel Management Process,* Houghton Mifflin, Boston, 1964, pp. 71-72.
3. Lester, R.A., *Manpower Planning in a Free Society,* Princeton University Press, Priceton 1966, pp. 4-5.
4. Patten, T.H., *Manpower Planning and the Development of Human Resources,* John Wiley & Sons, Inc., 1971, pp. 31-33.
5. Eric. W. Velter, "The Nature of Long Range Manpower Planning," *Management of Personnel Quarterly*, Vol. 3, No. 2, Summer 1964, pp. 20-27.
6. Joel Seidman, *American Labour from Defence to Reconversion,* University of Chicago Press, Chicago, 1953, pp. 152-172.
7. Dale, Earnest, *Management: Theory and Practice*, McGraw Hill, New York, 1965, p. 349.
8. Garth L. Mangum and Arnold L. Nemore, "The nature and Functions of Manpower Projections," *Industrial Relations,* Vol. 5, No. 3, May 1966, pp. 1-2.

5

HUMAN RESOURCES DEVELOPMENT PLANNING

"Time misspent is not lived but lost." —*Thomas Fuller*

"Zeal is fit for wise men but is found mostly in fools."
—*Ancient Proverb*

Coping with changes in market conditions, rising expectations of employees, development in technology and changes in management systems have necessitated increased emphasis on Human Resources Development (HRD). Knowledge in HRD is widening with many organisations setting up separate HRD departments and experimenting with different mechanisms of HRD. Based on the HRD experience of several public and private sector organisations, we discuss below how organisations can strengthen their HRD functions.

Human Resource Development is the process of helping people competencies. In an organisational context HRD by which the employees of an organisation are continuous and planned way to: (i) acquire or sharpen capabilities required to perform various functions associated with their present or expected future roles; (ii) develop their general capabilities as individuals and discover and exploit their inner potential for their own and/or organisational development purposes; (iii) develop an organisational culture in which supervisor-subordinate relationships, team work and collaboration among Sub-units are strong and contribute to the professional well-being, motivation and pride of employees.

HRD process is facilitated by mechanisms (instruments or subsystems) like performance appraisal, training, organisational development (OD), feedback and counselling, career development, potential development, job rotation, and rewards.

Employees are continuously helped to acquire new competencies through a process of performance planning, feedback, training, periodic review of performance, and assessment of the developmental needs, and creation of development opportunities through training, job rotation, responsibility definition, and such other mechanisms.

HRD Climate

A development climate can be considered as consisting of a culture which supports:

1. **Autonomy:** Employees have some freedom to act independently within the boundaries of their role/job.
2. **Trust and Authenticity:** Employees, departments, and groups trust each other and can be relied upon to do whatever they say they will do.
3. **Confrontation:** Employees face problems and issues without hiding or avoiding; them for tear of hurting each other.
4. **Collaboration:** Employees collaborate with each other and have a feeling of belonging to the same family and working for a common cause.
5. **Proactivity:** Employees are action-oriented, willing to take initiative, and show a high degree of proactivity
6. **Openness and Risk-Taking:** Employees feel free to express their ideas and the organisation is willing to take risks, experiment with new ideas and new ways of doing things.

Any organisation that would like to be dynamic and grow can do so only by making its employees dynamic and growth-oriented.

Steps for Strengthening HRD

1. Prepare a plan identifying the HRD mechanisms envisaged for implementation and their interlinkages
2. Assess the nature of the HRD needed—short-term and long-term—in the context of the organisation's history and plans
3. Assess the organisation culture and prepare an implementation strategy and plan
4. Choose one or a few subsystems for implementation suited to HRD needs
5. Decide the structural aspects of the HRD function
6. Get the time commitment of top management and of concerned line managers
7. Come to a clear understanding with top management and line managers about expected outcomes
8. Identify internal resources and task forces; get the help of external consultants, if necessary to augment and strengthen internal resources
9. Develop internal monitoring mechanisms. Build in periodic-review and renewal mechanisms
10. Be sensitive to suggestions of line managers and keep them informed.

Assessment of HRD Needs

An organisation may think of strengthening its HRD function for one or more of the following reasons.

Increasing Production

An organisation going for massive production increases without significant diversification in its products or services would need to focus primarily on role clarity, performance appraisal, and performance counselling. This is because no new managerial tasks are involved. Only the complexity of the tasks handled by supervisory and managerial categories may increase. In addition, new positions may be created at supervisory and managerial levels. To maintain the motivation of staff, it is necessary to appraise the potential of employees and develop them to handle higher level positions. As target orientation is required, it may be necessary to develop performance appraisal systems that promote role clarity, joint discussion of tasks and targets, performance analysis, and problem-solving. A good performance appraisal along with increased support from the training function may help.

Diversification

If an organisation is having diversification plans, new tasks and positions are likely, to be created. In, such a case, a carefully worked out potential appraisal and development system helps identifying and developing new competencies in existing staff. Such a potential development plan needs to be supplemented by a good training strategy and a development-oriented appraisal system to train employees on the job. If diversification activities require internal recognisation, a series of role clarity exercises with OD interventions supported by performance appraisal systems will be helpful to develop the employees.

Coping with Changed Conditions

Another situation such as, when market conditions change— for example from a sellers' to buyers 'market of when more competitors enter the market. The employees will be required to perform some new tasks without any substantial change in their positions or roles. They may be required to take more initiative, become more competitive, quality conscious, or service-minded. Such organisations have to reorient their staff through well-designed in-company programmes along with a development oriented appraisal system that promotes new tasks to be performed by the staff, new values, and attitudes.

Organisations that have reached a saturation point in their growth are likely to face problems of declining motivation, frustration, and alienation in their staff. In such organisations overemphasis on performance appraisal and training may some-times add to frustration. Programmes have to be designed specially to contain frustration. In such cases the concept of development takes new dimensions like motivation development and frustration management. Process-oriented OD interventions, job enrichment exercises, reward mechanisms, specially designed training programmes on management of stress, management of frustration, and retirement planning may help. The HRD effort should aim at equipping employees with competencies to manage career frustration and enjoy work. Personnel and career counselling services are likely to be of use. Performance appraisals should promote open communication and provide opportunities to dissipate tensions.

The first step in planning an HRD strategy is to decide the HRD needs of the organisation. The needs should be both in terms of immediate and long term goals of the organisation.

Preparing HRD Plan

With changing conditionsthe HRD needs of an organisation also changes. Various types of organisational needs described above may change, resulting in the need for change in HRD interventions. Therefore, it is useful to prepare a comprehensive HRD plan for the organisation. Such a plan should indicate the HRD mechanisms to be used, their, phasing, their interlinkages, and, expected synergistic effects. An HRD plan has to tackle the following questions:

— What subsystems should HRD begin with?, (e.g. performance appraisal or training or OD)

— Should there be a separate HRD department or should

HRD be a part of the personnel department? If separate, then what links would it have with personnel

- — What mechanisms should be used to monitor HRD implementation
- — What should be the budget for HRD?
- — How much of line managers, time is to be devoted?
- — What results can one expect from HRD?

Choice of Subsystems

HRD mechanisms are many; not all of them need be introduced or strengthened simultaneously. Starting with emphasis on one or two mechanisms is particularly important for organisations that are newly starting the HRD function or HRD departments. As most of the HRD mechanisms require time commitment of line managers, starting too many subsystems simultaneously distracts the organisation from its main tasks. The mechanism to start with is determined to a great extent by the HRD needs of the organisation outlined earlier.

Organisations Culture Assessment

To determine the subsystem of HRD that one should start with, it is useful to assess the HRD climate of the organisation. Simple questionnaires, like that for HRD climate survey developed by Centre for HRD at Xavier Labour Relations Institute (XLRI), are helpful in finding the HRD weak spots in the organisation.

Structuring the HRD Function

HRD function could be handled by personnel, training, and OD managers provided:

(a) they have a separately allocated resource

(b) they have sufficient time to develop for the HRD function

(c) they are acceptable to line managers

(d) these managers are positioned at higher levels in the organisational hierarchy

(e) they are charged with specific responsibility to facilitate and strengthen the introduction of HRD

(f) they have HRD and process facilitation competencies

(g) they are perceived as broadbased in their function.

In case, if a separate department is being established, its linkages with personnel and other related departments (e.g. training, if it is separate) needs to be worked out. If there is a training function it should be integrated into the HRD department as training becomes one of the core activities of the HRD department. When such new structures are created it is equally important for the organisation to develop integrating mechanisms. Most organisations use a director level, vice-president level, or at least a general manager level functionary as in charge of personnel and HRD. He performs the integrating role.

Committed Top Management

HRD efforts are not likely to succeed unless top management is highly committed to HRD. The chief executive should have a high degree of commitment to HRD and should be willing to communicate it to the employees. Investment in developing people is not likely to give short term and visible results. This is because managers require time to acquire new competencies— specially managerial, human, and conceptual skills.

Howsoever excellent a performance appraisal, training, counselling, OD, and job rotation system one may have, higher order competencies like initiative, dynamism, leadership, and organising capability get developed only over a few years. Such changes may not be visible in one or two years except to a very sensitive eye. Therefore, the chief executive Should indicate his faith in HRD. He should have patience and a sensitivity to notice growth in his employees. If a year after introducing a new appraisal system or training, the chief executive starts commenting that he is seeing very little change in employees, the HRD staff gets demoralized and wrong signals are read by line managers. Of course, this does not mean that top management should not ask for some results. In fact they should ask for results from the HRD department and senior line managers but the results should be asked in terms of competency development, problem-solving, and climate creation rather than in terms of balance sheets.

Involvement of Line Managers

HRD implementation is ultimately in the hands of line managers. Line managers work under pressure and are constantly under tension. Whether the organisation is growing or plans to grow or is going through a crisis, line managers are under pressure. Due to the innumerable environmental constraints, management systems while systematising most managerial processes also add to the pressures of line managers. In such conditions, it is understandable if a line manager does not perceive his job as also involving the development of his subordinates. He tends to forget this role in the process of meeting day to day task requirements and crisis situations.

Clarity about Expected Outcomes

Employees have a habit of expecting all their problems to be solved when a new technique or system is introduced. The managerial class is no exception to this.

Therefore, it is important for the HRD department or those in-charge of implementation to state clearly the expected outcome.

Hiring Consultants to Strengthen Internal Resources

Organisations introducing new HRD mechanisms a few years ago depended very much on outside experts as consultants. Today the situation has substantially changed. The body of knowledge on HRD was also small. Today plenty of experiences are available to learn from. There is a new professional body called the "HRD Network" started by HRD managers of a few organisations to share their experiences continuously and to learn from each other. With these developments, most organisations today are in a position to strengthen the HRD function on their own. Even so, some organisations may find it useful to associate an external consultant to give a fresh outlook, to keep communicating developments elsewhere, and to guide line managers.

Monitoring Mechanisms

Periodic review of the progress made in developing human resources can be useful in rectifying mistakes, if any. The task forces appointed to implement HRD should review the progress once a year. Progress could be assessed using questionnaires to survey the perceptions of line managers. If a HRD climate survey is conducted in early stages of introduction, periodic repeat surveys may indicate effectiveness of the HRD instruments implemented. Such reviews can also take the form of departmental meetings, review workshops, or specially commissioned studies by internal teams or outside experts.

Summing Up

An institution builder makes himself dispensible by building the competencies of his employees. He uses the time released by becoming dispensible to deal with external environment and create opportunities for the organisation to grow and make an impact. HRD instruments can aid him to move in this direction. Small investments in HRD with the commitment of the chief executive can go a long way in building the competencies of employees and a healthy and dynamic organisational culture.

6

HRD: TRAINING AND DEVELOPMENT

Recruitment of a new worker is an important aspect of employment. The acceptance of a job is the entrance into a community in which the worker, as a social being, will seek human satisfaction. This satisfaction depends very much upon his being accepted therein. This is a two-sided process. On the employer's part the applicant has to be turned into a worker who is satisfied with his job and the environment. On the other hand, a worker has numerous questions in his mind. His doubts and fears need to be clarified.

To achieve this dual aim a defined practice based on experience, imagination and sympathy is needed. It is a mistake to leave the worker to know and clear his doubts at the working site. The prospective worker should have required induction when a job is under discussion or soon after his selection. A worker may first come into contact with the receptionist or employment exchange officer when he calls at the employment office. How well he is received will affect his attitude to his engagement at the time and during the years of his employment. He will appreciate courtesy in manner, reasonable clarity and orderly arrangements throughout.

When he has been engaged, the employee must be clear as to when he is to begin work and to whom he has to report.

A written form of engagement containing these particulars avoids misunderstanding. A printed statement describing the ways of the firm and the rules governing the work and the workers should be given to him or explained by someone who is conversant with these rules. A brochure setting out the most pertinent work rules and explaining any important points of conduct, especially where personal safety is concerned, may be printed for this purpose underlining the more important rules.

Training the Workers

Approach to the Problem

The training of workers can be viewed from three angles:

(i) It is the follow-up of selection. Selection is only the first stage in the fitting of the individual into his job. The selector needs to keep in touch with those he has selected. On the one hand, he may check his own techniques and success and, on the other, he may ensure that individuals are rightly placed. Business sense calls for an adequate opportunity to be given to all suitable persons selected for employment to learn their jobs.

(ii) It is the process of learning applied to the work room. Different people learn in different ways. But learning can never be effective unless carried out in a systematic manner. The training of workers, therefore, in common with all other kinds of teaching, must take into account four factors: (a) the learner, (b) the jobs to be taught, (c) the trainer and (d) the methods to be used.

(iii) It is a means adopted for achieving greater competence. The trained worker is on the road to becoming more efficient. Unless an absolute limit of capacity exists, no employee of any grade, whether manual, clerical or executive, can fail to benefit from training programmes.

The problems which arise in the process of training will be revealed in consideration of these points.

(a) The Persons to be Trained

The persons to be trained may belong to different age-groups having varying capacities to work. They may be adolescents coming fresh from school or entering somewhat later into an industry. They may be men or women—single or married—from different walks of life and occupations. Some will be suitable only for unskilled work, though a few may be good material for training in relatively skilled occupations. Workers in these situations present many kinds of human problems. They will react differently to the same methods of instruction and will learn at varying levels. As such, they call for individual treatment from the trainers.

(b) The Job to be Learned

The jobs may be just as varied as the capacity of the learners. They may be unskilled, semi-skilled, or even relatively skilled. They may be mass production or repetitive work. They may be complicated, or may be simple and easily learned. Simplicity must not be overstressed, since few establishments keep an individual continuously on one sub-divided element and, therefore, instructions must cover the job as a whole. Moreover, a person learns better if his interest has been stimulated by showing him where he fits in the chain of production.

(c) The Trainers

Proper training involves competent instructors. The steps necessary to procure competent instructors are:

(i) Selection of persons who know the processes and jobs thoroughly; can express their ideas clearly; can describe movements accurately; and are patient and tactful with slow learners.

(ii) Introduction of these persons to the methods of teaching. This would include a statement of the general laws of learning and common maxims governing good teaching and at times detailed methods for instance showing how to pack, or to assemble the particular parts on which they are to work.

(iii) General instructions to the instructors in such matters as the source and supply of materials; the inspection of finished goods, time and motion study; costing and planning; wage calculations or any matter on which questions might be expected from the trainees.

(iv) Clarification of their own views on the human problems of training to bring these views into line with the company's policies.

Methods of Training

Training methods vary from the unorganised system of learning from working colleagues to more systematic methods of instruction.

(a) Learning by "Exposure"

This is still the most common method, especially in smaller factories. It is a costly and ineffective system subject to criticism on two grounds:

(i) From the angle of the worker. Proper teaching takes time and will reduce output where trouble is honestly taken in training another.

(ii) From the psychological standpoint this method may not be unsatisfactory. It is learning by imitation, or more precisely, by "exposure" to the example of another. Even though it may be a good model, imitation can never be perfect and instruction in such circumstances proceeds by the correction of errors. However, mistakes at times imprint themselves on the memory and, become part of the unconscious, show themselves in bad working habits. Their eradication takes a long time and makes learning by "exposure" costly.

(b) Systematic Training—Vestibule School

The main characteristic of the vestibule school is that it is in a separate room which may be part of the work room but still distinct from it. Its location and setup give it certain advantages.

(i) The pupils can be brought more into the classroom spirit; they will be less distracted and consequently the teacher will be able to use his specialised skill more effectively.

(ii) Emphasis can be put on good quality production and attention given to the weak points of the pupil. This can encompass temperamental and other qualities, and the school be made a helpful bridge between the class room and the factory.

The vestibule school has its removed, if it is to be made effective.

(i) The atmosphere may become unreal, work being made too simple and difficulties removed too fully.

(ii) Speed may be, sacrificed and a tendency to "slow motion" set up.

(iii) The school may become an end in itself, with the result that the pupils experience a sense of shock when they are transferred to the workroom.

These drawbacks, however, will be obviated if certain steps are taken.

(a) To avoid unreality, the work in which pupils are trained should be production work.

(b) Some firms insist on quality first and speed up to the standard later:

(c) The danger of the school being an end in itself can be removed by arrangements which give it an acknowledged, place in the factory organisation.

Training in the Workroom

Training in the workroom takes place under normal conditions of work. It is organised instruction for which generally the foreman is responsible even if he does not teach the workers himself. The workroom has its disadvantages as a place in which to teach and learn. The distractions of the bench are considerable.

Concentration of attention is not easy and amidst the prevailing noises, the worker may fail to catch the full meaning of important instructions. A plus point is the environment in which the learner has ultimately to work. His discouragement will, on the whole, be less if he faces the working difficulties during learning. Here the discipline is that of the foreman rather than of the teacher. If the disadvantages of the workroom can be reduced, it can prove better than any other method.

Training the Office Staff

Whether government or private efficiency of an office, depends on the quality of the staff. While the sense of responsibility and loyalty to an organisation is important, it cannot be a substitute for good knowledge of the job techniques and scientific methods of operation. For example, an employee, howsoever loyal and devoted to an organisation, cannot handle the correspondence work effectively if he lacks good expression. Similarly, an employee having years of experience may not be able to use the latest techniques if he is not familiar with them. The administrative offices where, on an average, an employee is paid many times more than a factory worker, can run economically and efficiently only when they are managed properly.

Among the four 'M's of management—men, money, machine and materials — it is the men who are most important for offices. While devising a training programme for office staff, several factors have to be taken into account. Individuals differ in their capacity, to works intelligence and basic aptitudes. The potentiality to grow is also not the same in all employees.

Even in the best managed organisations, not all people joining at the level of assistants and clerks will retire as directors or senior executives. The requirements of the office and the role that it plays in the whole set-up of business are also to be kept in view while training its people.

Some of the important factors which influence training programmes are as follows:

Age

Naturally, all men have a similar capacity to grow in age but not with age. Those who adjust themselves to the changes taking place in their environment, equip themselves with the latest knowledge and techniques and apply their minds for improving their efficiency, rise in life. Not all employees take the initiative themselves to learn continuously and advance. People in the older age group, therefore, need training as much as those in the younger age group. It is necessary to wipe out orthodox practices, procedures and methods in an organisation and introduce scientific ones. Training young minds is easy as they have no inhibitions. Old employees do not forget the past so easily.

Academic Qualifications

Men who have acquired knowledge through university and college education cannot be bracketed with those who have not. It is not only a question of faith in the degrees and diplomas of our universities but also a fact that experience is a substitute for academic qualification only in a limited sense. Trainees are, therefore, to be grouped according to their academic achievements. Sometimes, even among the trainees who hold the same degree, distinction may be made on the basis of their levels of achievement. A trainee, with a brilliant academic record may be more receptive and may take less time in grooming than one with poor academic records or one who is an easy going person. In making such distinctions, however, the basic aptitudes and interests of the trainees have to be left in view.

Aptitude and Interest

Employees differ in their basic interest. Some are very intelligent but not hard working, while others may be hard working but lacking in intelligence. It is the job of the trainer to make people feel interested in their work and to improve their knowledge. The likes and dislikes of the trainees for particular jobs, responsibilities etc., cannot be ignored. Some employees like table work, while some others may have more interest in liaison, coordination and field work. Moreover, training can remove certain misgivings or orthodox beliefs regarding the nature of a particular job and thus create an interest in the employees.

Job Requirements

An office is primarily a means to attain the objectives of business. It is the nerve centre of modern organisation. There has been tremendous increase in the volume of office work in recent years because of governmental regulations and publicity work. The kind of work done in all offices is basically the same, i.e., processing the information for efficient coordination of production distribution and financing of merchandise or services. This processing of information involves four steps: communication—written and oral; summarising operating results, record keeping, systematising and cost reduction. The scope of training, and curriculum are determined to a certain extent by job requirements. For better-communication, proficiency in a language is a must. Proficiency may be attained through regular courses, guided readings, film shows, writing contests, etc.

The organisation may have to build a library of its own. For improving record keeping, training in modern methods of accounting and costing is essential. The efficiency of an employee can also be improved by training him in the modern methods of office communication, set-up and administration. General awareness of the economic and social environments, governmental regulations and technological change should be included in the training curriculum for all types of staff.

Training of Management Trainees

The future of any corporation depends largely on the availability of the right type of executive personnel at the right time. Well trained managers are hard to find and the business houses cannot always approach the open market for their requirements. They have to develop a cadre of professionally qualified people to man the key posts in the future. Moreover, each organisation has its own culture and requires the people who not only accept it, but are also acceptable to it. The expanding business organisation with progressive outlook, therefore, regularly recruit management trainees while smaller organisations do so infrequently, depending on their requirements and resources.

A well planned training programme for management trainees is a must for developing the creative faculties of trainees and orienting them to the practical aspects of administration. The training should start with an orientation programme in which the trainees are introduced as the executives of the organisation and acquainted with its policies and programmes. They are familiarised with the past history of the organisation, its activities, its work and offices, its products and its people. They may be addressed by some of the company executives, and provided with the company's balance sheet and other printed information giving details about the organisation. They may also be sent on visits to different factories and offices of the company. The familiarising programme should be as informal as possible. It is also desirable not to create any false impression in the minds of trainees in the beginning to avoid frustration in the future. The trainees should be placed on the job after their orientation. The rotational job programmes are considered best for them.

They may be placed under the supervision of the heads of selected departments for stipulated periods, so that they learn the rudiments of the job from the very beginning. It would be desirable not to treat them as "crown princes" while they are on the job training. They can learn something from the man at the lowest ladder also. While in the job, the trainees should be carefully observed and their activities should be analysed. Their observation power and ability to do the jobs and adjustability are on test. They can also make their contribution to the administration by bringing new ideas and new procedures against the established ones, some of which may have become obsolete. The trainees may also make unbiased comparison of the working of different departments. During the entire period of training, each trainee may be placed under the care and guidance of one senior level executive.

The system of understudy may be adopted for making one executive responsible for the development of one trainee. Even when the trainee will be on the job in other departments, his supervisor will have remote control on him. This system, however, works well only when realy competent people are made supervisors who may compete among themselves in producing the best manager out of the trainees rather than creating their henchmen.

Group discussions, seminars and case sessions are important means of developing the trainees. In a group discussion trainees get an opportunity to improve their power of expression and deliberation and also their knowledge by having a cross-section of opinions on different issues. Their personality also comes into play in such meetings.

The trainees may also be sponsored for short-term seminars and courses organised by management institutes so as to gain from the experience of experts in the field of management. During the entire training period good reading material should be provided to the trainees. Selected articles on management, technological advancement, industrial, commercial and social problems should be distributed among them from time to time. A reference library should also be built for them. A system of reward and recognition may also be introduced to motivate trainees. The training period may be reduced in the case of trainees who show an outstanding ability to learn and develop in a short time. The provision of benefits such as housing for trainees may prove to be a strong motivating factor.

During group discussions and seminars the trainees may be asked to preside over the meeting in rotation. The company's regular interview boards may allow one of the trainees to sit as an observer. A system of counselling should be built for the trainee whose performance may not be up to the mark.

In the organisational hierarchy the number of positions at the top level are limited. At the lower level, the aspirants for middle and higher positions are many. The middle managers find themselves in a dilemma in a situation like this. Only a few of them get the opportunity to rise to senior positions. Some may manage to retire honourably. The fear of being dismissed looms large on the heads of the remaining. They are supposed to make place for those on the waiting list at the lower level and the new entrants from outside. Openings outside may not always be very bright for them. What should they do? Who is responsible for all this? What should the organisation do for them? These are some of the problems which have attracted the attention of management scientists recently.

The factor which render shelf-sitters incompetent are mainly physical, mental and social. Most of the middle management positions are occupied by people of the middle age group. They may lack the energy and the enthusiasm which are the characteristics of young managers. They may lack dynamism also. Their habits acquired rightly or wrongly, characterise them. In their effort to please bosses or suppress the juniors they may overact. Family responsibilities and financial burdens may compel them not to take risks and accept challenge. Those who reach middle management positions at a very young age may feel frustrated early if they are not wanted at higher levels when they wish. Those who reach middle positions at the fag-end of their career after having served for the most part of their lives in low positions, are natural shelf-sitters.. They deem it an honour to retire on these positions. The bureaucratic organisations in particular are full of people in the older age group on middle managerial and administrative posts. They carry the virtue of indecision, redtapism and strict adherence to certain false notions and principles.

The organisation's inability and incompetence which develop a band of shelf-sitters may be both due to inner constraints and managerial policies. Few organisations can afford to give opportunities to all middle personnel to adorn the top positions. Those who are close to the top bosses go up, while others have to sit on the shelf or go out. Defective manpower planning and recruitment practices are also responsible for the growth of self-sitters. Sometimes the large organisations create well "paying positions which have little-real function and fill real jobs with totally unqualified people. The beneficiaries of the largeness then become the victims of it.

The organisation can help considerably in preparing the shelf-sitters for better careers outside. It may introduce a plan under which a manager earns educational credits or "green stamps" (based on the length of service in lower and middle management), which he can cash in to pay for academic courses that prepare him for better job opportunities outside the organisation. The shelf-sitter should be given an indication in advance that he would not be considered for better positions so that he may use his "green stamps" to forge a second career and avoid demotion and stagnation. The expenditure on a plan like this would certainly be less than that in retaining the unwanted shelf-sitters. On humanitarian grounds too it is desirable to equip an employee better for a career outside if there are not enough openings within the organisation.

The emphasis in the "green stamp" plan is on increasing the educational qualifications. The success of the plan, therefore, depends on the availability of educational programmes and job opportunities based on these programmes for middle managers.

The "green stamps" may also reduce the chance of becoming shelf-sitters. Fresh training may change the attitude of the manager, develop his skill and knowledge and he may become useful to the organisation. Thus the plan may "tackle a real problem" and contain a hidden bonus for corporations as well as potential shelf-sitters.

Training the Executives

The executives who are responsible for getting things done through the efforts of the people need training for several reasons. Majority of them occupy senior positions by virtue of exercising responsibility in less senior roles in the same organisation. By winning the confidence of their superiors on account of hard work and loyalty, many of them may have easy access to higher positions, even though they may be lacking in some of the skills for such positions. The specialists and technical personnel who rise to executive positions need more general managerial abilities. Moreover, their specialised knowledge may go out of date.

Social Changes

The executive of today is living in a dynamic society. The last few decades have witnessed changes of far reaching importance in our social and community structure. The contributions of psychologists, sociologists, anthropologists and other social scientists have enriched management science in many ways. Some of the presumptions regarding human nature and the methods of dealing with men have gone out of date. An old fashioned executive may take pride in talking of the good old days when his orders were respected like the command of a military officer and followed unquestioningly and ungrudgingly. The new generation is different. Men in industry are better organised and conscious of their rights and privileges. The officers come from different strata of society. Senior positions are no longer restricted to a particular class of society. The changing social structure demands greater awareness on the part of executives.

Identification of Training Needs

It is debatable whether the executive's immediate superior should identify his training needs. The superior's superior may be more suited to identify such needs because of his position as he may be free from some of the apprehensions which the immediate supervisor may have. A scientific system of appraising merit is of great help in identifying training needs. The areas of deficiency may be located and it may be ascertained as to which skills require improvement and in which areas acquisition of new skill and knowledge is essential.

A generalist managing a technical section may be better equipped if he acquires some technical knowledge. A highly qualified technical lesson may lack in some of the important aspects of human relations. An executive may be good at work but poor in communication, while another may be good at communication but poor at execution. A non-financial executive dealing with financial matters may face some difficulties which can be overcome by acquiring basic knowledge of finance management. A controller of stores having no knowledge of modern inventory control methods and techniques may find himself handicapped in dealing with critical issues involving stores.

Role of the Training Division

While it is basically the responsibility of the bosses to identify training needs, a training division can be of great help, both in devising the appraisal system and locating the areas of deficiency.

Organisation of internal training programmes and sponsoring of outside seminars and courses are the responsibilities of the training division. Internal training should be informal in nature. Executive club/study circles may be formed to have informal gatherings. Experts from cross-sections of society may be invited to address the groups from time to time. Business games, case sessions and, film shows may also be organised for the groups. Such meetings may foster better relations among the executives and may be informative and stimulating to them.

Seminars and Outside Courses

Executives usually welcome participation in conferences and outside courses for several reasons. They are free from office routine for some time. Their performance is not watched by the bosses. They get an opportunity to meet their counterparts in other industries and exchange ideas with them. They can participate in the deliberations of the conference/seminar with an open mind. They also get a sense of achievement as participation in an outside course amounts to improvement in their qualifications.

An advanced course/seminar for senior level executives should have the following characteristics:

1. It should be of short duration, since the executives are mostly busy with heavy responsibilities, and long-term courses are not likely to attract many.
2. It should be organised at a place fitting with dignity, status and convenience of the executives.
3. It should be drafted in such a way that the executives with different academic backgrounds may find it easy and interesting.
4. It should be drafted with instructional methods including lectures, case sessions, group discussions, business games, selected readings, conferences, project reporting, films and audio-visual aids. Group discussions and case sessions are preferred the most.
5. The faculty should consist of both the professors and the business executives.
6. The number of participants should be limited in order to develop inter-personal contact between the participants for a smooth running of the courses.

Training must be a continuous process. The changes in attitudes, behaviour, leadership style and other individual traits do not come in a day or week. The desired results in this direction are achieved gradually. The effects of company training programmes and participation in outside courses and seminars are to be judged over a period of time.

A regular training programme linked with a scientific system of merit appraisal and counselling goes a long way in improving, organisational efficiency.

7

CONCEPT OF MANPOWER INFORMATION SYSTEMS

Manpower Information System is also essential for any manpower planning activity. In a climate of rapid environmental change and increasing awareness that the only real competitive advantage is to be found in the quality of our people and how well we use them, an effective manpower information system is an essential aid.

Output

An analysis of intended uses and required outputs is a useful starting point in designing what the system needs to be able to do and assessing the adequacy of your existing system. The general objective will be to ensure that the system can provide the necessary information, in a form that can be integrated with any other business data, which means that it has got to be comprehensive, up to date, accurate, and probably not stand-alone.

Beyond that, the objectives become specific to applications. With most database systems, there are facilities to pull out any of the data and present them in whatever form is required, but this sort of friendliness does vary. Applications should, therefore, be detailed. An analysis of the elements (modules) offered in proprietary systems, which we can presume have responded to market demands, show that the main thrust is to provide facilities for basic personnel administration, with strong links to payroll and pensions administration.

The outputs required from such suites can be listed, and then the precise formats determined so that these can be programmed. Using the same example, the outputs might be:

- salary listing for salary review purposes;
- salary review analyses and summaries;
- salary drift/wage drift, by grades, plants, etc.;
- compa-ratios movements in average salaries by grade;
- performance rating analyses;
- grading distribution by grade within departments, divisions, etc.;
- salary distribution salary scatter within grade salary ranges, by occupation group, or area, or division, etc.

Inputs

A large number of personnel departments still retain those large green folders containing all of the paperwork associated with each employee, although it may now have a printout of his current computerised record. When a new employee joins an organisation, he or she normally completes an application form, which provides the basic data for opening an electronic record. It is the electronic record which is updated and which is always used, with fresh data added on job and remuneration changes, training courses attended, and changes of dependants, addresses, etc. From time to time, a printout of the current record is sent to employees to enable them to confirm that all is correct. This initiative invariably flushes out a collection of acquired qualifications and domestic changes but it should not flag errors in job titles, salaries or other internal data, which should be fully up to date at all times.

The data elements in a complete manpower information system are likely to include the following information.

1 Identification

Surname and forenames

Works or computer reference number specific to the individual

2 Other Personal Information

Address (including postal code) and telephone number

Next of Kin

Date of Birth

Sex

Marital Status

Nationality and work permit detail, (if relevant)

Race for analysis of race-relations practice

Registered disabled person (if relevant)

Trade union membership number

Relative within company

3 Organisation Locations

Company or division within group

Location

Department

Cost centre reference number

4 Occupation History

Earlier Work experience

- Employers
- Positions held

- Dates

Date of joining:

- Details of broken service if relevant
- Recruiting source
- Status of employment: full-time, part-time, temporary or contract
- Positions held within company:
  - — dates appointed
  - — job titles and departments
  - — job grades
  - — occupation codes

5 Salaries and Benefits

Salary history

- Basic salary or wage
- Dates and amounts of changes
- Reasons for changes
- Planned next change amount and date

Hours

- Normal hours
- Overtime paid/not paid
- Shift work

Bonus

- Supplementary payments, etc.
- Bonus scheme eligibility
- Amount, timing and criteria

Benefits eligibility/awarded

- Holiday entitlement
- Company car
- Medical insurance
- Company loan, etc.

Pension scheme membership

- Scheme
- Date joined
- Normal retirement date
- Life assurance cover, etc.
- Link to pensions administration system

6 Performance and Potential Assessment

- Most recent performance data
- Most recent data covering potential
- Psychological test score, results and dates

7 Qualifications

- Level (GCSE/A level/degree/doctorate)
- Field
- Specialist/professional
- Apprenticeship, etc.

8 Training Received

- Training courses attended
    - — internal/external
    - — level of course
    - — duration
    - — dates

- Training planned

9 Competencies

- Competencies required in present job
- Personal competencies
- Competency requirements
- Language skills

10 Development Plans

- Career moves possible

  Planned next move (if relevant)

  — position

  — occupation code

  — job Grade

  — timing

11 Succession Plans

- Entries in succession plans

12 ***Medical History*** (confidential — restricted access):

13 ***Absenteeism***

14 ***Overtime / Shift Work/Part-Time Work***

Depending on the system in use, some of this information may need to be coded to facilitate analysis. This is an easy enough task when the range of choice is limited, but increasingly difficult as the complexity of data increases. Academic qualifications can be covered through a series of steps or decimalising the breakdown. Elements such as current job and, even more so, past experience, offer an enormous range of choice and coding difficulty. In some systems, this entails the creation of one or more separate files which subsequently need to be linked to the main file for some analyses.

Job Coding

Job information is difficult to use unless it can be translated into some form which computer logic finds easy to handle for analytical purposes. The best way of doing this is to use a numerical coding system, in which each job has a unique number, and the numbers form a logical pattern.

The Department of Employment's system known as Classification of Occupations and Directory of Occupational Titles (CODOT) has, since its design in 1972, provided a comprehensive, even complex, system of classification to cover all occupations found in Great Britain. This system lists about 3800 separately identified occupations, each of which is defined so as to cover five basic components, namely:

1. A short statement of the occupation's essential characteristics,
2. The main tasks normally carried out;
3. Common specialisations and additional tasks;
4. Additional factors that are important when considering employment in the occupation;
5. Other alternative titles for the occupation.

The 3800 occupations are grouped at three levels, namely:

1. 378 Unit groups of occupations which share similar tasks;
2. 73 Minor groups, combining Unit groups which are related in terms of work performed;
3. 18 Major groups, combining Minor groups into comprehensible main headings.

Two other standard classification systems that have been in general use are the classification of Occupations (C080), as developed in 1980 by the Office of Population Censuses and Surveys, and the International Standard Classification of

Occupations (ISCO), as developed by the International Labour Office and daring from 1968.

Whilst these three systems of classification (CODOT, C080 and ISCO) have certain similarities, the government departments that made full use of them, both in Britain and in the European Community, have sought to harmonise occupational and other statistics to international standards. The result of this has been a major revision of ISCO (ISCO 88) which came into general use in most European countries during 1990/91. In Britain, a major revision of both CODOT and CO80 has produced a new British standard known as Standard Occupational Classification (SOC). This appeared in 1990 and is available from HMSO in three volumes. It is closely compatible with the European standard ISCO. 88.

Those companies that are considering introducing a standard classification system to their own job structures would do well to look at SOC. It would make for easier comparison with future British and European Community statistics.

S.O.C retains certain features of its "parents'. The 3,800 occupations defined by CODOT are now analysed into 371 Unit Groups, 77 minor Groups and 9 Major Groups. The decimal notation is retained but only to three levels instead of the four levels used by CODOT. As a result, the classifications do not provide the same level of detail as CODOT and may, therefore, be more manageable for companies to use themselves. An example of the less complex nature of SOC is the personnel Officer referred to above.

It would be possible, if you so wished, to introduce your own fourth digit to differentiate between Personnel Officers and Industrial Relation Officers. This method of coding also means that it is not possible to have more than nine sub-categories of each group. As a result, the digit '9' is retained as a 'bucket[1] at each level of classification for groups that are 'not elsewhere classified'.

SOC may be less comprehensive than CODOT in the coding structure it provides. It does, however, provide a consistent and sensible approach to the classifications at each level, based on two key criteria — (1) skill levels and (2) the nature of work activities.

> **Skill Levels**—where appropriate the classification takes into consideration either the level of formal qualification required for an individual to be recognised as fully competent in the occupation, or the period of training/experience required to do the job competently.
>
> **Nature of Work Activities** — the classification considers any or all of a number of aspects of the work, including the materials handled, the type of tools and equipment used, etc.

What is generally not considered by the classification at each level is the status of the person doing the job. So, for example, the jobs of trainee clerk, clerk and office supervisor all appear under the same classification code. There are, however, some specific exceptions to this in the classification of managerial levels.

The definitions at the Unit Group level comprise:

A brief statement of the job content;

Typical entry routes and associated qualifications;

Tasks;

Related job titles.

Job Information

It is important that job information used for analysis should be properly maintained and up to date. Usually, this requirement is tied in with job analysis and grading for remuneration purposes, highly motivating when keeping things up to date. Without job information, recruitment would be virtually impossible, training would have no target, salary administration would have no basis, organisation structure and manpower planning would have no solidarity.

Job information refers to the essential data on the job which identify it and set it apart from other jobs. The information we require will concern its duties and tasks, the associated authority and the potential effect of action taken, responsibilities for assets and personnel, plus the specific objectives or standards to be achieved and the resources and time allocated for the purpose. The ideal incumbent will also be specified.

It is not particularly difficult, within any company, to find out what jobs people are holding. It is known who is called chief engineer and who is called a billing clerk and so on, but job titles do not tell the whole story. For example, the managing director of a small organisation may operate his own production machines and type his own letters, while a technical assistant known to the author had considerable responsibilities for a costly research and development programme.

Proper job information is, therefore, essential. It has wide ranging applications, including job grading, salary administration and recruitment, and will often have associated relevance in the training and personnel development fields, or for organisation planning.

Job Families

Any form of job coding or job evaluation is likely to make use of the way in which jobs tend to cluster into families, i.e. families of associated jobs such as chemical engineers, or cost accountants. In job evaluation, it is not difficult to judge;

the relative values within a series of accounting jobs, or within a group of development engineering jobs, but it is rather more difficult to tackle the evaluation of an accountant in relation to a design engineer.

Some job evaluation processes totally avoid the question of comparing jobs in one family with those in another, limiting their results to series of job family based but, otherwise unrelated, structures.

Equally, within job families, movement between jobs is relatively straightforward, because job holders have related skills, while transfers between families are more difficult. Within a job family, the knowledge and skills required are closely related common scales of education and training exist— so that the flow of people between jobs is predictable.

The relevance of job families here is that they provide the parameters for many career flow structures, and also that they define limitations on manpower supply, particularly for categories in short supply.

Taking flow structures first, flows are likely to be reasonably free within a job family. Accountants are able to move to more senior accounting jobs as they acquire experience, but would face some difficulty moving into a different stream. Even within accounting, they would have difficulty in moving from the mainstream to one of the subfamilies of specialisms such as those in the treasury or corporate tax office. Appointments in each subfamily are likely to be filled by other specialists from the same subfamily but possibly from a different company. The flow follows family lines.

When a shortage occurs usually as demand rises it would be useful to examine a nationwide flow chart, which operates in the same way as in company pattern. There is an attempt to pull through a larger volume of people at particular levels than the input flow and development activity can generate, and the how fails to respond.

The response to the recent shortage of corporate lawyers has been a great increase in the intake at the bottom end, speeded up development, many promotions made too early and exceptional pay for younger people. The activity is so specialised that it is not practical to draw in people with different training and experience, the only source being from the ranks. This possibly has resulted in larger numbers choosing to study law at university. It will be a number of years before the situation balances out. It is possible that, at an interim stage, the heavy wave of fresh people will result in an oversupply at middle levels, leading to reductions in intake at the bottom.

Analyses of various categories show the same pattern national shortage is followed by a surge of supply at university entrance and company intake levels, and a subsequent reaction against oversupply which clogs career flows. Chemical engineering is another good example from the past. One finds trained chemical engineers in a great variety of different careers, having been frustrated in their initial ambitions through being part of an excess supply.

In examining the structures of career flows, a knowledge of job families is relevant, together with an understanding of supplementary skills necessary to facilitate movement across boundaries. For example, there is frequently a flow from research and development into sales and marketing, and to manufacturing; this flow is aided by product knowledge. These flows can be assisted by specific training designed to provide the additional skills relevant to planned future transfers.

Competencies

A number of organisations have developed the practice

of building up a profile of required competencies for each job, particularly at more senior levels. If the same competency profiling is applied to all existing personnel, there is a basis for matching people to jobs for short-listing candidates. The *Executive TRACK* system offers this facility, leaving open the selection of competences to be used as there appears to be an infinite variation judging from individual company lists. As discussed elsewhere in the book, the identification of competencies needs to be based on the priorities in the business concern, on corporate culture, and on the actual use of terms within the company, to ensure that the words used are meaningful to the users. They do not need to convey anything to outsiders.

The value of this process for analysis depends on the relevance and accuracy of the selection and definition of competences; of the identification of competency requirements in individual jobs; and of the assessments of the strength of competences in individuals. In my view, much of the work done so far has lacked precision, although the quality of analysis is improving steadily, so that this will be a valuable aid by the mid-1990s.

Lack of precision appears to result from attempting to define universal management competences. This can be overcome by shifting the focus to specific groups of jobs, possibly in one job family, but perhaps best by concentrating on a functional unit of organisation. Within a department which has a specific commercial purpose, the success criteria guide analysts to the specific areas of competence which are critical. These are not universally required of every person, but need to exist in balanced quantities for overall team efficiency. When the same competences are sought within the team staff itself, it becomes possible to identify the competences requiring strengthening, which in turn will upgrade departmental effectiveness.

Executive TRACK has the capability to store competency information relating both to the attributes of individuals and the requirements of positions. The information can be generated from a variety of sources, such as assessment centres, psychometric tests, performance appraisals and skills audits.

Once held within a database, the competency data can, for example, be used to identify training and development needs or to perform candidate searches. Competency profiles are used to help identify a short list of international candidates managers who may be suitable for a specified position and to generate a best-fit score of their attributes in comparison with job requirements. It is possible to use fairly complex mathematical techniques to generate a score.

This may involve weighting the individual calculations, or identifying critical and non-critical factors, or both. However, this example uses the simplest method, which is a straightforward running total of the differences between the position requirement scores and the individual competency scores. It is important to note that one would never make a candidate selection decision based on this information alone. As well as other, more objective information which can be used to identify suitable staff, the final decision will almost always be based on traditional methods.

The value of using competency profiles is principally to narrow down the range of candidates (assuming that a wide range of candidates is available) and to focus attention on the relative merits of each one.

Manpower Models

A large number of off-the-peg software packages are available for various aspects of manpower planning. Some of them perform narrow, specific functions and some assemble substantial data banks for major analyses associated with business options.

The most useful form of model for most manpower planners is one which can respond to 'what if?' questions, or which will enable a series of assumptions to be balanced in relation to each other to provide a desirable end result.

As with any computer application, the machine will do only what it is told. Therefore, the purpose of a model needs to be determined, and the calculations which it is to make must be programmed precisely. Even a complex programme is basically straightforward provided that the workings of the manpower situation are understood and the flows within it have been quantified. If the patterns can be written down, they can certainly be programmed. This in greatly simplified form. Every company organises its people planning process according to its needs, and some use only parts of a total system. It was noted earlier that some of the standard Packages address only limited aspects, and the market for such software demonstrates that interest is restricted in some areas.

The key issue in any planning is that the elements should be complete and fully integrated. In a full manpower model, the essential elements would need to be covered comprehensively, and the time and volume links between the sets of data would need to be interlocked.

The model used earlier in the chapter contained the basic elements, and for practical purposes would be quite adequate. Additional elements bring the model closer to real life. When building a statistical model, judgements have to be made, at a number of points, on the implications of, say, a culture shift, a change in employment legislation, or the quantification of performance standards. For some purposes, a very large-scale and complex model may be developed, but its accuracy will only be as good as the accuracy of its elements.

The impact of a strategy along these lines can be calculated quickly, with subsequent medication of the assumptions until it appears achievable and likely to meet the target levels. Communication of this strategy may well be somewhat restricted, but it provides key guidelines to all key managers and HR. people for achieving the change.

Personnel Software

A number of database systems are available to assist managers in the planning and administration of human resources. The most popular ones tend to be PC based since they provide the user with greater independence, control and flexibility than has previously been possible using corporate mainframe systems.

An exhibition called Computers in Personnel, sponsored by the Institute of Management Studies, included 58 exhibitors. The bulk of the systems on offer were basic packages associated with personnel, payroll and pensions administration, and absence control. Others had particular applications to the administration of large volume recruitment.

Relatively few packages have sufficient scope to be relevant here. One that does and is now, perhaps, the most widely used is *Executive TRACK.* It is supplied in the UK by Business Advisers Limited. *Executive TRACK* is primarily designed to enable human resource managers to store, organise, analyse and present the information required for management development, career, succession and manpower planning. It was one of the first packaged systems to become generally available for these applications and has since been adopted by over one thousand companies world-wide. *Executive TRACK'S,* developers have successfully refined the system over the years, based on the practical experience and input of many of the world's leading companies.

The ability to analyse the inventory in almost any conceivable way is made possible by such a system, and these analyses provide vital data for projecting future manpower availability, an essential ingredient in manpower supply planning.

Business Advisers Limited also develops and supplies the *HRI View* statistical report generator which has been used to prepare many of the tables in this book. *HRI View* effectively combines an ad hoc reporter and a spreadsheet in one package which manpower planners can use to produce statistical reports from employee and job information held in *Executive TRACK* databases, or link to business planning data. A further package, *Corporate CHARTER*, enables information to be prepared in the form of organisation and succession charts.

8

HUMAN RESOURCE FLOW MANAGEMENT

"The most men often give the best advice." —*Philip J. Bailey*

"A wise man adapts himself to circumstances as water shapes itself to the vessel that contains it." —*Chinese Proverb*

Basically, Growth requires recruitment, development, and promotion of an expanding pool of competent managers and technical specialists in organisations. Increasing competition in mature industries may require fewer employees—ones with a different mix of talents, capable of responding to different environmental demands. Strategic decisions concerning how an organisation will respond to its environment must be matched by equally strategic decisions concerning how the organisation will manage the flow of employees. Not having the right skilled workers or managers when they are needed can seriously undermine the success of strategic business choices. Just as damaging is a surplus of human resources which can be costly to the corporation and potentially damaging to the sense of well-being of employees.

Unfortunately, the problem of ensuring that the right people are available is not merely a problem of forecasting personnel requirements, difficult as that task is. The availability of needed talent is also a function of the organisation's capacity to attract, keep, and develop the people it needs. These tasks require that management adopt a social capital perspective. Employees are treated as investments which if properly supported and developed can yield a long-term stream of benefits to the organisation, not as variable costs to be hired when the organisation is growing and laid off when the organisation is retrenching (though clearly cost effectiveness must be of continuing concern).

An organisation's continually changing requirements for types and numbers of people are sometimes poorly matched with concurrent employee needs for stability and opportunity. The objective of human resource flow policies is to meet the corporation's current and future force requirements and employees' career needs at the same time. Obviously, these objectives may be in conflict. Unions are often formed as a result of conflict between employers and employees about these very issues. So, human resource flow policies must reflect management's values about the relative importance of organisation and employee needs.

Managing Flow Perspective

We are suggesting that flow policies can be approached from the point of view of the *individual* employee and of the *organisation.* Increasingly, these policies must also reflect the interests of yet another stakeholder: the organisation's host *society.* These interests are imposed upon the organisation through government legislation and regulatory agency policies concerned with such matters as employment, promotion, termination, and retirement. Though the role of government differs from country to country, its involvement reflects the fact that corporate policies on human resource flow have a profound effect on people's economic and psychological well-being, and therefore have an effect on the economic and social well-being of society as a whole. Thus, flow policies can be examined and evaluated from the following three perspective.

(1) Individual Perspective

The term "career" is too often seen as applicable only to

the lives of managers and professionals, and not to the lives of nonexempt white- or blue-collar workers. Typically, the term connotes upward mobility and aspiration. From that perspective, an assembly line worker or a restaurant waiter is not thought of as having a career. As a result, corporations focus career development efforts on their professionals and managers, while ignoring blue-collar workers. Since human resource management applies to *all* employees, a broader concept of career seems to be in order. From this broadened perspective, careers may be viewed as "a series of separate but related experiences and adventures through which a person, any person, passes during a lifetime." Careers can be long or short, and an individual can pursue multiple careers either in sequence or at the same time.

In this sense, the concept of career becomes a shorthand notation for a particular set of activities with a natural, unfolding history—involvement over time in a given role or series of roles. An individual attempts to gain control of these "separate but related" experiences so that they fit an emerging self-concept (self-perception of unique competence and values). At the same time, that self-concept is progressively shaped by work and family experiences.

Central to this broader definition of careers is the component of identity. As Erik Erikson has said, identity is never gained once and for all, but is achieved throughout life. Individual careers develop from an interaction between the competencies and career goals an individual brings to the organisation and the work experience the organisation provides.

To the extent that the organisation provides opportunities for the individual to use and develop his or her personal competence while moving through various jobs, functions, and levels, the individual will grow and experience career satisfaction. Organisations may respond to strategic requirements for certain skills by altering the types of opportunities they provide. For example, a strategic decision to develop more generalists rather than functional specialists must be accompanied by human response policies that provide opportunities for and encourage multifunctional experiences. Multifunctional experiences also provide an opportunity for individuals to clarify their career goals and to decide whether this developmental direction is personally satisfying.

Each career experience leads to a new understanding of self as new successes or failures redefine how individuals see themselves, their potential, and their limitations. Each experience therefore reshapes an individual's career aspirations. Major failures can lead to career crises which arise from job choices that do not fit the individual's core competencies and personality.

Understanding and managing a process that avoids major failures but makes possible personal learning and growth is critically important if organisations are to develop their employees while at the same time giving them career satisfaction. It is generally accepted that the more control an individual has over career choices, the more the individual is likely to choose a career path that fits his or her core competencies and values, thereby ensuring satisfactions and growth.

Historically, individuals had little control over their life's work. Career choices were determined by one's station in life, one's family, and one's society. Most organisations gave employees little control over their careers, preferring to make placement and promotion decisions without consultation. It has become increasingly clear that this practice cannot continue, given the desire and power of today's employees to exert more control over their careers.

The wider concept of career implies that it is impossible for organisations to apply a single definition to what desirable career development is. For managers and professionals, it may be an opportunity to develop and advance, though advancement may be defined differently by an engineer and an achievement-oriented business school graduate. For many blue-collar and white-collar workers, employment security and stability may be more important, while security may be of lesser importance to managers and professionals. Assessments of career needs are complicated by changes in career aspirations that take place throughout the life of a person.

It is important to note that employees' perspectives may differ between cultures. Do Japanese workers have different career needs with respect to rapid promotion and do they desire less control over their careers than American workers?

(2) Societal Perspective

The social perspective can be said to impose itself on the organisation in one of three ways: through the shifting values of the work force, through the impact of outside institutions, and through regulation and labor union policy.

Complicating the problem of managing human resource flows is an apparent shift in social values away from a view of work as the single most important aspect of life, and toward a view that work is only one of many facets of life. Strategic decisions concerning internal movement and career development of employees can no longer be made without taking into account this growing emphasis on both self-development and family development. Employees no longer automatically accept job assignments that their employers consider important for their development if these assignments conflict with personal and family needs. Similarly, blue-collar workers no longer accept as given the fact that they must and should work overtime. As educational levels increase, blue-collar workers may grow dissatisfied with the same routine job for the duration of their careers. Flow policies that give these workers opportunities for career progress will become more important. These trends probably apply most to economically developed countries where standards of living are high and security needs have been met, freeing individuals to seek fulfillment of other needs.

The emergence of knowledge workers as a growing proportion of the work force makes organisations increasingly dependent on educational institutions. Not only do these institutions control the number of people that will be available to corporations, they often create and define career paths in society through program decisions. These institutions also socialise people within particular career paths. The expectation and values of the students they turn out may or may not mesh with organisational realities. When they do not, frustration and turnover are often the result. The current shortage of engineers in high-technology companies, and the frustration of pharmacists with their roles in large pharmaceutical chains are only two examples of such mismatches between the programs of educational institutions and the needs of business. An interactive process between educational institutions and business is required so that educational institutions will be able to shape and modify their programs to business needs so that corporate human resource flow policies will mesh with educational realities.

Government bodies and labor unions are increasingly responding to the needs of people for employment security. There is growing research evidence that the unemployment that results from corporations that treat labor as a variable cost creates psychological stress and social dislocation. Losing one's job can increase family problems, endanger emotional health, and increase the likelihood of alcoholism, drug abuse, psychiatric disorders, cardiovascular disease, and even suicide. In Europe, high severance pay requirements and other legislative restrictions on an employer's freedom to terminate employees have resulted, in part at least, from an awareness of such negative costs. Under the restraints imposed in many European countries, managers will have to manage in a way that stabilises employment and offers more security.

As the cost of termination increases, or the flexibility of management decreases—through either government legislation, social pressures, collective bargaining agreements, or explicit unilateral policy decisions by employers—management will have to give increasing attention to deciding which employees to hire in the first place and efforts to train, retrain, or otherwise develop their already available human resources. This has been true for some time in Japan, where approximately 30 per cent of the work force—those in large corporations—have lifelong employment, and it appears to be the direction in which some United States corporations are also going. On the other hand, legislation is often used to open career paths that historically have been available to only a privileged few. Workforce, welfare, and unemployment policies affect the careers of people and the supply of people available to firms. Similarly, licensing and standardisation of occupations in various states and industries affect corporate selection and training policies. In the United States, equal opportunity legislation has and will continue to have significant effects on hiring, internal placement and promotions, and termination practices.

Selection methods and performance evaluation systems are being challenged in the courts on the grounds of their validity and objectivity. Class action suits, brought against companies by the Equal Employment Opportunity Commission (EEOC) on behalf of groups of employees, can end in settlements worth millions of dollars. The most celebrated of these suits, involving the EEOC and AT&T, ended in a consent decree costing the company 33 million. There has also been an increase in the number of lawsuits that employees in the

United States are bringing against corporations claiming unjustified discharge.

The emergence of legislation and regulations governing flow policies reflects the recognition by society that corporate actions have pro-found effects on the well-being of people and society as a whole. Lay-offs, for example, have economic consequences for the communities in which they occur. Because of strong family and community ties, some unemployed workers will remain in their city or state instead of looking for work in other sections of the country.

Layoffs thus often place the greatest financial burdens on the communities that can least afford to carry it. When social and government agencies are burdened by the social and psychological problems resulting from layoffs, *all* citizens end up paying an economic and social price. Though less dramatic, flow policies that do not allow personal development and utilisation of employees' talents also reduce the quality of life and have social consequences.

(3) Organisational Perspective

Because of the relatively slow pace of change, skill requirements did not change much over time. Many jobs such as accounting or management had not yet emerged as professions, and there were few technical and professional schools to supply needed talent. Government was relatively uninvolved in employment issues. There was also a large supply of labor willing to move from agriculture to the factory and office. All of these factors have changed. The emergence of the knowledge workers in the labor force, rapid changes in technology and business practices, the increasing need for generalists, more complex organisations, the emergence of minorities and women, mobility of the work force, and the greater involvement of government have made the management of human resource flow policies a more important consideration. Rapid change can result in costly excess work force, while rapid growth can mean insufficient workers. The unavailability of an experienced plant manager is clearly as critical to the success of an operation as the unavailability of capital resources.

From the organisation's perspective, effective flow policies should lead to the following results:

1. Development of people needed to staff the organisation in the future.
2. Availability of the right number of personnel with the needed mix of competences in the short and the long term.
3. Employee perception of opportunity for advancement and development consistent with their needs.
4. Employee perception that selection, placement, promotion, and termination decisions are fair.
5. The lowest possible payroll and people-processing costs possible to meet the objectives above.
6. Employee perception of relative security from termination due to factors beyond their control.

It should be understood that policies concerning recruitment, selection, promotion, and termination of employees are the means by which institutions can shape a philosophy of management; they are often the implicit means by which a corporate culture is formed. Not only do people become socialised through their experiences with flow policies, they also come to recognise the qualities of behaviour that will be rewarded with promotion, and they come to form views about management's concern for their well-being.

Policies, Systems and Practices

The Human resource flow must be done within the constraints imposed by social institutions, and with the well-being of society in mind. At best, managing human resource flow is imperfect. Some people will always be insecure or unhappy with the opportunities afforded them. Every organisation has considerable "noise levels" associated with these issues. Similarly, the best personnel planning process may not deliver the people needed by the firm because employees do not grow as expected or because business projections do not materialise. However, major discontinuities can be avoided and employee satisfaction can be increased by more deliberate planning and examination of particular policies, practices, and systems and their relationship to each other.

1. *Managing Inflow*

Recruitment decisions about where and how to recruit can have an important impact on the composition of the work force, its ultimate fit with the corporation's needs and culture, and employee turnover. These decisions affect all of the four Cs: competence, commitment, congruence (conflict), and cost effectiveness.

Problems in recruiting, particularly for certain professional and technical talent, arise when educational institutions fail to yield an adequate flow of qualified graduates. The recurring shortage of engineers, for example, results from fluctuations in the supply of engineering graduates and experienced engineers (which in turn are related to demographics and past educational patterns), and from fluctuations in the overall demand for engineers. The organisations can apply the following methods an adequate supply of talent:

1. Human resource functions can provide schools, particularly schools from which they recruit, with forecasts of future personnel needs.
2. A decision to locate facilities in the proximity of educational institutions that graduate people with the

needed competencies or in industrial centers that already employ such people can increase the availability of talent.

3. Corporations can use visits and summer jobs as a way of identifying talent and involving students early in their schooling, perhaps several years before they are ready to enter the job market.
4. An organisation that develops a good reputation as an employer in such areas as employment security, compensation, employee relations, and opportunity for challenging work and growth can increase its capacity to attract recruits.
5. Corporations can develop their own educational institutions, as Wang Laboratories and General Motors have done.
6. Corporations can establish ongoing relationships with universities by assigning key executives to coordinate recruiting and by donating time, equipment, and people to those schools.

Recruiting Effectiveness Criteria

The first and more obvious reason is that recruitment seeks to provide the organisation with people who have the talents needed to achieve strategic goals. But recruitment will also have significant impact on long-range employment stability and turnover. Employee turnover is both disruptive and costly. It is well known that the most important reason for turnover within the first several years of employment is mere expectations, and these disappointments are often a function of the recruitment process itself. Managers motivated to attract scarce talent tend to discuss only positive elements of the job and company while glossing over less attractive realities. They do not help the prospective employee to assess realistically the fit between personal skills and goals and the job and the organisation. A more open process of communicating organisational realities would yield employees who were satisfied with their careers. New hires would be more highly motivated to adapt themselves to organisational realities. The likelihood of fit in expectations, skills, and core values between themselves and the organisation would be higher because more self-selection would take place. Some companies have found that training line managers to conduct recruiting interviews can improve the effectiveness of recruitment.

Obviously, the recruitment and "joining up" process should not be looked at only from the point of view of its impact on cost effectiveness and congruence or conflict. Recruiting can be an important strategy for shaping the culture of the organisation. It is at the time of recruitment and entry into the organisation that an implicit "psychological contract" begins to be formed between employee and organisation. Prospective employees receive many signals about what the company expects, just as company recruiters make many judgments about the suitability of the prospective employee with the organisation. Understanding these transactions can help general managers understand the culture of their organisation. Reshaping these transactions; can help them develop their organisation in desired directions. For example, the choice of which managers in the corporation will recurit and make final selection decisions will affect who enters the organisation, and what their competencies, predispositions, values, and expectations will be. It is for this reason that key line managers often involve themselves in recruitment interviews.

2. *Internal Flow Management*

Once employees have been recruited, their flow through the organisation—transfers, job assignments, promotions, and demotions—must be managed so that their competence is developed to meet corporate needs, while at the same time they satisfy their own career aspirations. The velocity of personnel flow, the assessment and measurement of performance effectiveness, and the development of employee skills and competencies are the key considerations in this regard.

Velocity of Personnel Flow

Velocity may be examined for horizontal movement (lateral transfers) and vertical movement (promotions). It varies widely between different employee groups in the corporation. Historically, middle and upper middle managers have moved from job to job rather frequently; the average time in a job being as low as two to three years in some corporations. Among clerical workers or technicians, the average time in a job may be far higher, say five to ten years. Similarly, managers in mature industries are likely to be in their jobs far longer than managers in growth industries like high technology or health care. Finally, velocity for different employee groups will vary across time periods. For example, the postwar baby boom will lead to a large population increase in the 35 to 50 age category between 1980 and 1990. That increase will be accompanied by a relatively slower growth in middle management jobs, resulting in fewer opportunities and slower upward movement.

Notably, any given velocity may have positive and negative outcomes with predictable benefits and costs, and these must be balanced by the general manager. The important point is that velocity is part of managing human resource flow and it warrants monitoring. Naturally, flow velocities are sometimes beyond control of management—demographics, for example, will affect velocity. But managers make some decisions that have consequences for human resource flow velocities but are not immediately recognised to have such effects. Too often, market opportunities are considered far more important than human resource considerations in determining a growth strategy.

Decisions about how many employees are to be recruited each year also affect velocity, as well as the availability of trained personnel in the future. Uneven recruiting from year to year, often brought on by economic cycles, can force rapid movement and promotion for one cohort of entering employees and too-slow movement for another. Such uneven recruiting patterns result in an uneven supply of talent to replace retiring employees or feed growth. Companies with lifetime employment that promote only from within have learned that steady recruitment is necessary to assure a balanced distribution of age and skill in the work force:

In evaluating the strategic impact of velocity decisions, managers can consider the impact of their decisions on the following HRM out-comes:

1. *Competence.* A curvilinear relationship probably exists between velocity and the development of employee competence. That is, slow movement of personnel (laterally or vertically) is likely to result in too few opportunities for employees to broaden their skills and their perspective of the enterprise—that is, to develop as generalists. On the other hand, the type of very rapid personnel movement that is experienced in rapid growth companies can easily result in individuals progressing faster than their capacity to develop and demonstrate skills. The result can be failure for the individual (the well-known Peter Principle) and a resulting loss of investment by the company.
2. *Satisfaction and commitment.* Satisfaction of employees with career development will increase if upward mobility in the corporation becomes more rapid. Lateral transfers also seem to have a similar effect. These in turn are

likely to increase commitment to the organisation because employees see a bright future in terms of personal rewards.

3. *Congruence.* Slower advancement can lead employees to question the fairness of the decision-making process in the corporation. The consequence can be litigation by employees, particularly women and minorities. On the other hand, high velocity can be so demanding that quality of life suffers, particularly in relationships with family. Personal stress and higher divorce rates are not uncommon among employees in rapidly growing high-technology companies. Similar symptoms have been found among blue-collar employees in new plants that are attempting to increase commitment by having employees rotate jobs, take more responsibility, and assume accountability.

4. *Costs.* High flow velocities are more costly. An employee who has been on the job a short time is less effective. Also, the costs of training and transfers are high and getting higher.

5. *Motivation.* There is also a curvilinear relationship between velocity and motivation. Too many years in the same job will reduce motivation, as the challenge that comes from efforts to master a new task declines. On the other hand, insufficient time to master a task not only leads to the inadequate development mentioned above, but may prevent individuals from developing a sense of competence and a continued desire to achieve.

Employee Effectiveness

The management of personnel flow through the organisation requires continual judgments by managers about potential effectiveness of recruits and employees. Poor judgments translate into failure for the individual, immediate costs resulting from poor performance, and long-range costs associated with missed opportunities to promote employees who have potential. Too many bad personnel decisions can leave an organisation without adequate backup personnel to fill openings created by promotions or retirements.

The major problem in selecting and evaluating effective employees is the subjective nature of the process. Except for education, academic performance, and specific technical skills, it is hard to measure the characteristics that are assumed to be predictive of performance: motivation, cooperation, ability to make decisions, initiative, ability to work under pressure, capacity to develop, and capacity to supervise. Even when attempting to be objective about whether a candidate possesses certain qualities, a manager sees the candidate through his or her own personality, past experiences, and values. Managers tend to hire people in their own image. While such an approach may ensure smooth boss-subordinate relationships, it may not ensure effectiveness, particularly if the biases imposed on the selection process—temperament, dress, social mannerisms, etc. are not in actuality related to performance.

Since managers' values and predispositions are subtly shaped by the culture of the organisation, the potential for systematic bias throughout the organisation is high. One of the by-products of managers hiring in their own image has been systematic discrimination against minorities and women. Government has responded to this discrimination with legislation such as the Civil Rights Act of 1964, requiring employers to hire and promote women and minorities in proportion to their presence in the larger population. If they cannot do this, employers must prove that their personnel decision-making process is based on job-relevant selection criteria.

While some corporations have always had an interest in

developing good and fair selection and evaluation procedures, government legislation and the potential for costly court decisions have stimulated a wider concern about this problem.

Such influence can come through the participation of employees in the definition of effectiveness and through their direct involvement in evaluating prospective employees, peers, and bosses. Employee effectiveness traditionally has been defined and evaluated exclusively by management, but consultation with employees can give managers the opportunity to improve their own judgments with relevant information and improve employee perception, of fairness.

Except for some blue-collar, clerical, and technical positions that are relatively easy to define, insufficient attention has been given to identifying the requirements for job success. As a result, typical specifications call for certain academic standing and work experience. These specifications have the virtue of being measurable. Unfortunately, they may not be relevant. Most selection processes, particularly those for higher-level jobs, tend to be based more on general parameters and subjective assessments than on defined characteristics that are assessed with objectivity.

Effectiveness, particularly in managerial positions, is also a function of the organisation's culture. Over time, many characteristics and ways of doing things come to be valued by the organisation and are implicitly or explicitly taken into account during selection and promotion processes. General managers must attempt to define as explicitly as possible what individual characteristics are valued. Personnel specialists can help by researching the characteristics that distinguish effective and ineffective performers as defined by judgments of the corporation's managers. This research process makes it possible for managers to examine these characteristics for their relevance to business strategy and organisational effectiveness and helps them identify irrelevant biases or important omissions. It allows top management to determine if their philosophy is adequately represented in personnel decisions and to take appropriate action if it is not. Organisations that rely on a strong culture of shared traditions and beliefs for achieving employee commitment must be especially concerned about selecting and promoting individuals with characteristics that fit that culture. Such organisations can sustain their culture only if they maintain a fairly high degree of homogeneity of values. They are, therefore, likely to emphasise personality and management style as significant dimensions, perhaps more than technical skill.

Of course, by doing so they may discriminate against certain employees, and take the risk that their biases violate legislative guidelines or society's values. So far, little has been said about results—sales, costs, profits, market share, number of units produced, etc. —as a criterion of effectiveness. This is not because we believe that the attainment of results is irrelevant, but because results are not the *only* criterion of effectiveness, even when they are espoused to be the primary criterion for promotion and compensation decisions.

When first introduced, quantitative measures of results were thought to be the way to make performance evaluations more objective. However, such measures do not always reflect important dimensions of performance nor are they always within the control of employees. Thus, "process" dimensions of effectiveness are often introduced in personnel decisions. Furthermore, the accomplishment of results at one level is not always a good predictor of whether an employee will be able to function effectively at higher levels in the organisation.

Individuals who achieve results *and* exhibit the behaviours, attitudes, and characteristics that experience suggests are effective and/or that managers believe to be effective are clearly effective performers and possess the potential to rise in the organisation. Individuals who do not obtain results and do not fit are rarely retained by organisations because they do not appear to have the potential to succeed. It is the individuals in the other two quadrants who present dilemmas for organisations. Those who do not achieve results but do fit behaviourally are sometimes promoted well beyond their level of competence. Organisations that attempt to identify high-potential employees early in their careers are subject to this error. These individuals may be promoted so rapidly on their *assumed* potential that they never master either the business management or technical task. On the other hand, some employees are not promoted despite a consistent record of results because they are not judged to possess the skills required for higher-level positions and/or because they do not fit the culture. For example, some successful plant managers or successful deal-makers in banks do not understand how they could have been passed over for promotion, given their job performance. What they do not understand, and what has not, been made explicit by their organisations, is that certain behavioural skills and personal styles are as strategically important to the organisation as are quantifiable and measurable technical skills. Because they do not know what these behavioural skills and style characteristics are or how strategically important they are relative to results, these individuals are unable to develop them or make the decision to seek other employment—an argument for explicitly defining and communicating behaviors associated with effectiveness.

If behavior is to be a criterion, attention must be given to the question of fairness as viewed by employees. Employees who do not believe that the criteria being utilised are relevant will either leave the organisation or protest by seeking legal redress or union protection. In the past, management has dealt with this problem by commissioning personnel research studies to establish the objectivity of effectiveness criteria. But this approach still leaves the power for defining effectiveness with management. An alternative approach may be to allow employees more influence in selecting managers or peers as a way of giving them influence in the definition of effectiveness. Peer ratings, which have been shown to be good predictors of effectiveness, probably gain their validity because peers possess information about each other that superiors may not possess. Some of the most innovative work systems in the United States involve members of work teams in the selection of new employees, although getting employees to rate their peers is difficult and requires extraordinary maturity and interpersonal competence. Employee task forces may be involved in defining effectiveness for their group, department, or plant, creating the standards that will guide personnel decisions in the organisations as a whole. Employee influence in defining effectiveness can only work, however, if employees and management share common goals.

Evaluating Effectiveness: Organisations face two sets of evaluation problems: evaluation of *prospective* and *of current* employees. Even if effectiveness has been adequately defined, managers must still assess the extent to which individuals possess certain characteristics. The most common methods for doing this are the employment and performance appraisal interviews. Because both methods have been shown to be subject to bias, they have been supplemented with other methods:

1. Structured interviews.
2. Interviews or performance evaluations by multiple managers/ evaluators.
3. Paper-and-pencil tests of ability, intelligence, personality, and interest.
4. Checklists of derived characteristics as guides to the employment and performance appraisal interview

5. Internally administered assessment centers and performance tests that ask individuals to perform tasks under simulated conditions.
6. Clinical assessments by psychologists or consultants.

These methods structure the assessment process so that information gathered is more reliable (less subject to errors in measurement) and more valid (the information is relevant and predicts effectiveness with greater accuracy) than is the information collected in employment and appraisal interviews alone. The predictive power of these additional assessment techniques is established by one of two types of validity studies. Either the characteristics being measured have been shown to be correlated with the present performance of current employees (concurrent validity), or scores on tests or evaluations are correlated with later performance on the job or advancement in the organisation (predictive validity). Another method for determining the validity of an assessment procedure is to examine whether the knowledge and skills being assessed represent adequately the actual content of the job (content validity). These methods of validation have all been subject to challenge in the courts. Of the three methods, content validity is most likely to be upheld by the courts. If more than one of the approaches to validation described above have been used, the organisation's assessment methods have generally been upheld.

Some companies use these methods to help evaluate the potential of existing employees, while others may attempt to increase objectivity (validity) through multiple appraisals, checklists of relevant characteristics, and the use of in-depth clinical interviews by psychologists or personnel specialists. Self-selection by prospective and present employees is a method that is underused by corporations. If employees are informed candidly and in some depth about the characteristics that are required for success, they will eventually select jobs or career tracks that are realistic given their talents and aspirations.

General managers need some familiarity both with the general concept of validity and with the specific applications within their organisations. More structured and well-researched methods of assessment can improve the organisation's probability of selecting the right people for specific jobs when effectiveness has been defined. What is less clear is the impact of these methods on the relationship between the individual and the organisation.

Do applicants or existing employees who are subjected to the various impersonal selection procedures resent them and, as a result, decide to go elsewhere? If so, what kind of people are alienated by these procedures, and how do they differ from those who are not? Would an emphasis on self-selection as opposed to formal selection procedures demonstrate an organisation's commitment to informed choice and self-control over career? If so, how would this emphasis affect who decides to take a job and how that individual subsequently relates to the corporation? These are all questions that general managers, as well as testing and measurement staff specialists, must weigh. The challenge to managers is to take advantage of available measurement and testing technology, while not losing sight of its effects on how recruits perceive and later relate to the organisation. The companies most successful in their use of sophisticated assessment methods have usually avoided using results in a rigid manner. It is important to recognise that the more openly and regularly assessment results are discussed with inside or outside candidates, the more trust candidates have in those results. Evaluations of employee effectiveness and potential are usually performed by supervisors and then used by management to make personnel decisions.

An enormous amount of time, money, and energy has gone into the development of different performance appraisal systems. While improved appraisal systems may better reflect job content, successful implementation still rests largely with the managers involved in the process. And a significant number of managers resist evaluating their subordinates. When controls force them to evaluate, they provide ratings of questionable validity. In response, some corporations have adopted forced distributions in rating employees. Quotas mandate a fixed percentage of employees that will be placed in each of the rating categories from poor to excellent. This type of forced distribution, however, is resented by managers and subordinates alike. It has the potential for damaging the self-esteem of individuals, particularly since studies have shown that a disproportionate percentage of employees rate themselves as high performers. Research evidence and experience suggest that managers assign more accurate performance ratings when those ratings are not used to make personnel decisions and/or when they are not made available to subordinates.

Because evaluations of performance are a matter of judgment, managers are naturally concerned about negative impacts on pay, promotion, and job security. They also prefer not to discuss these ratings with subordinates, because they do not want to damage relationships. If they have to justify the ratings or if personnel decisions about pay, promotions, or terminations are to be made as a result of their judgments, ratings tend to be less valid.

Employee Career Development

There are two major concerns that a human resource flow policy must address when considering ways of managing internal flow. The first, addressed above, is the question of how to define and evaluate performance effectiveness.

Consistent with the social capital perspective of HRM, we would also suggest that internal flow policies need to address the matter of employee and career development. After selection, employee development is one of the key methods available to corporations for ensuring the mix of skills needed to be competitive in the future. It is a form of investment which is directly related to the corporation's capacity to be flexible and adaptable to changes in its environment. In short, employee development is a key strategy for organisational survival and growth.

Far from taking a coherent and strategic approach to employee development, many corporations engage in scattered, uncoordinated, or even inconsistent developmental activities that are poorly suited to the developmental needs of individuals or to the corporation's strategic needs. Training departments plan programs and market them internally in accordance with their perceptions of developmental needs, which do not always coincide with the strategic goals of the company or individual employee needs.

Employees are often transferred or promoted on a timetable dictated by organisational needs, not by their own readiness. Participation in a training program may not coincide effectively with the need for education created by a job transfer or promotion. Assessment, feedback and counselling methods are rarely coordinated to maximise the learning and development of the individual. This lack of coordination between centralised practices and the individual's needs can reduce development.

The challenge, then, is to *stimulate and guide* an essentially individual developmental process in a way that is consistent with corporate needs. Some corporations operate with few centrally planned career development programs, while others have chosen to centralise and control the process to the detriment of individual choice, growth, and career satisfaction. The most effective approach is for general managers to create a context that encourages employee development in directions that meet corporate needs but does not overdetermine the speed or direction of any given individual's development. Through this process, employees can determine if they have the core competencies to master the task. If they do not, they obtain feedback that the career directions chosen are not the right ones. If they do master the new experiences or jobs, the resulting sense of accomplishment confirms the direction chosen and sustains it as long as the experience continues to be satisfying. Employees must, of course, stay in their jobs long enough to obtain closure, to see the results of their efforts.

This cannot happen when the velocity of movement in the firm is too rapid. It should be clear that the most important developmental experiences are job and task experiences. This fact is not always reflected in the mix and sequence of developmental tools used by corporations. Education and training, which are not always sequenced to complement a special assignment, seem to work best when job experiences have motivated an individual to learn needed knowledge, and when they are accompanied by feedback on performance and counselling from a respected supervisor. When the slow growth of a firm precludes promotions as a means of providing growth experiences, job enrichment—the redesign of work to include more responsibilities—is used increasingly to stimulate development and reduce costs. Enrichment is usually applied to traditionally fairly narrow blue-collar jobs, but it can also be applied to middle management, where too many jobs and levels have increased costs and reduced opportunity. Lateral transfers are another method of providing an opportunity for development and growth short of promotions. Organisations need to inventory these tools in order to make them known to managers and to develop plans to help managers use them.

Education programs are easier to inventory than job enrichment programs, which is why they are more frequently used. But it is the competence of supervisors in performance appraisal, coaching, counselling, modeling, and supporting that is the key to a program's success. Therefore, if career development is to occur in an organisation, general managers must find ways to select, train, and reward so as to build these elusive developmental skills. Some corporations are supplementing the supervisor's role in coaching and counselling with a staff of personnel specialists trained in this task.

Career development workshops and assessment centers are also utilised to provide participants with a guided experience in exploring their interests and aspirations.

Probably the most important but underutilised part of the developmental process is follow-up. When developmental plans are created by a supervisor and submitted to the personnel department, it is essential that the company follow up to determine what the result has been.

Career opportunity information. In order to ensure that employee development is successfully meshed with an organisation's strategy, it is essential that the organisation encourage employees not just to develop, but to develop in directions required by that strategy. Are technical skills likely to become less valued in the coming years as compared with general management skills? Will the company be placing more emphasis in the upcoming years on the interpersonal and behavioural skills of its managers? Is it likely to need a more aggressive sales force? Will competitiveness hinge on low costs, efficiency, and productivity? It is not only important for organisations to be able to answer such questions, but the answers must also be *communicated* to employees.

Only through such communication will employees have some idea of what skills will be valued in the future and what experiences are considered important in developing those skills. To do this well, corporations should project the types of jobs and skills requirements they estimate will exist in the future given their business strategies.

Will the competitive edge in the future be obtained through production, sales, or technical work? What mix of skills is likely to be valued, to fit evolving corporate strategy and culture? Just as important, what have been the career paths to general management or technical management in the past? Estimates of future growth can never be totally accurate, but employees should be encouraged to think about what paths successful people in various careers have followed and how these paths might change in the future. Information can be disseminated through publications, training programs, and the audiovisual medium.

The career paths a corporation makes available to its employees have an important influence on the extent and nature of their development. One way to characterise career paths is in terms of whether they encourage functional or technical specialisation, or whether they encourage cross-functional mobility. Investigations of companies that have not adapted well to competitive pressures, those in the steel industry for example, show that these companies have developed few generalists capable of becoming general managers, product managers, or program managers. Individuals were brought in at the bottom of a function and promoted within it, causing them to retain a specialist's view. A strategic emphasis on adaptation to new competitive demands might suggest an emphasis on cross-functional mobility in order to break down barriers between functions, develop individuals who understand the views of other functional specialists, and develop employees committed to the solution of business problems.

In each organisation, there are some career paths that are more valued than others. The valued track can be managerial (referred to as cross-functional above), or it can be technical. Typically, managerial jobs are more valued for the status, power, and monetary rewards associated with them. Attracted by these rewards, individuals in technical or sales jobs often attempt to switch careers and seek managerial positions despite the fact that their skills and/or interests may lie in their technical specialties. A firm needs to examine the career decisions that its internal job market encourages to determine if these decisions are consistent with its strategy and needs for employee competence.

Conventionally, blue-collar workers and white-collar clerical and technical employees have not had much opportunity to progress to more challenging jobs. Locked into their stations, their on-the-job enthusiasm and capacity for learning and growth declines. In response, some companies have attempted to stimulate growth and commitment through job rotation or job enrichment. Others have designed skill-based pay systems that align rewards with learning and development.

Organisations also need to consider the opportunities for upward mobility, that they provide to blue-collar and white-collar clerical and technical employees. A two-class society has been created in many companies, lowering cooperation and commitment to common goals. The removal of artificial barriers to advancement such as the requirement of a college degree is one method of increasing employee competence and commitment. Other ways of increasing the corporation's human assets include providing education and training, and providing job experiences that allow lower-level workers to gain the knowledge, attitudes, and behaviour required to join the managerial class.

Career authority and control. There are three principal means by which the corporation can provide individuals with control over their careers.

First, an organisation can develop a cadre of *personnel development specialists* to whom employees may go directly to discuss their career goals and receive information about realistic career possibilities. These specialists typically are involved in helping managers find candidates for open positions, so they are aware of opportunities. They provide an employee with an alternate route for career management if his or her boss is ineffective or too controlling. But these specialists also serve the corporation, which means they play the difficult role of representing both employees and the organisation.

Again, employees can be asked to fill out an *inventory of skills and job preference,* which can be cross-referenced for use in job searches.

Finally, a system of *job posting* allows employees to apply for other positions in the company when they become vacant. An increasing number of companies are using this method in an attempt to give more direct career control to employees. It calls for employees to respond to announcements (postings) of positions and to be considered just as if they were external job applicants. The personnel department may screen applicants for a job before giving the hiring manager a list of potential candidates. The hiring manager interviews applicants, decides who to hire, and provides feedback to successful and unsuccessful applicants. Job posting has been adopted widely, particularly for lower-level jobs, because it appears to solve the problems of control. The courts and regulatory agencies such as the EEOC have looked favourably on job posting as in indication of affirmative action and nondiscrimination, one reason why an increasing number of corporations are adopting the system. However, job posting does not ensure fairness. In some cases, supervisors have decided who they want to hire before posting, making the interview a sham. Furthermore, the screening process is subject to bias. Finally, unless the company is willing to explain to employees why they have been rejected, the system may simply raise expectations and then dash them. Despite its weaknesses, job posting has potential for giving individuals some control over their careers, provided the corporation is open and willing to invest in the method by giving supervisors the proper training.

3. *Outflow Management*

A company may attempt to improve its mix of competencies rapidly by increasing the outflow of personnel through early retirement programs and/or layoffs of the lowest performers. Early retirement increases the percentage of younger personnel who management often believes are more flexible in adjusting to a changing business future than older, more entrenched employees. At the same time, personnel reductions allow for a rapid lowering of payroll costs, which can improve profitability in the short term. In the United States, this scenario has been used by companies in many industries as a response to recession and competition. Pressured by the quarterly earnings expectations of investors, corporate management has used work-force reductions as a major strategy for maintaining earnings and dividends expected by investors, stock analysts, and financial institutions.

Legislation in some European countries and a social contract between unions and management in Japan have placed significant constraints on layoffs in those countries. Some restrictive legislation on terminations and layoffs is also beginning to be seen in the United States, suggesting that American managers will find it increasingly difficult to use personnel outflow as a strategic response to competitive pressures. Individual rights and the welfare of society will become more important considerations. Under the Age Discrimination in Employment Act of 1967, as amended in 1978, older employees are protected from forced retirement prior to age 70. In some states there is no upper limit. "There is a tremendous increase in employee lawsuits, particularly over age, sex and race discrimination and unjustified discharge," says Robert Conken, president of the American Arbitration Association. These pressures will modify the policies of U. S. firms toward more caution in layoff and terminations, ultimately moving them closer to the full employment model.

The *central strategic dilemma* for managers is how to balance the needs and rights of employees for employment security with the requirements of the corporation to use personnel outflow as a means of cost reductions and renewal. Research evidence and experience demonstrate that employees who become insecure because of work force reductions are less productive and less committed to the organisation. The best tend to leave after the economy turns around.

On the other hand, unless corporations take extraordinary care in the selection, training, and internal movement of personnel, legislative barriers to outflow can erode competitive position. How can corporations and society obtain the benefits of employee security without incurring the costs of overstaffing and stagnation?

Lifelong systems guarantee employment only if performance is maintained. If performance declines, so does pay, and employees are pressured either to improve their performance or to reexamine their relationship with the company. Terminations occur for poor performance on a case-by-case basis and not when a recession and profit squeeze provide a convenient excuse. This policy requires continual attention by management to performance and a willingness to confront problems.

Atain if corporation cannot offer employment security to all of its employees, it may still choose to offer it to some of them. The number of employees is based on the lowest employment level economic circumstances are likely to force on the corporation. This policy does not deal with the potential obsolescence of the core group nor is it known what effects the policy will have on relations between protected and unprotected employees.

Downward and lateral career mobility. One means of achieving a better balance between required job skills and job holders without termination is to utilise downward and lateral mobility, particularly late in a person's career. A division manager may move down to head a function from which he or she came, or a salesperson who has been promoted to management may welcome returning to sales again if he or she is given proper status and recognition. Companies that deemphasise hierarchical position and emphasise professional competence as a source of power are more able to move employees out of managerial positions with dignity.

Early retirement. By offering special financial inducements, many companies have increased the outflow of personnel they consider unable to adapt to a realignment of the firm. Usually the inducement is retirement at an earlier age without a reduction in pension. The employee is able to retire at age 55, but will receive benefits he or she would have received at 62 or 65. The individual is then free to pursue a new career if he or she so chooses, and the firm can offer promotions to those they believe to be more competent to perform in the future. This is the single most popular option for managing outflow used today by American firms to revitalise themselves in the face of international competition.

Career renewal. Companies can encourage individuals to leave oversupplied positions and move to undersupplied positions through effective training and development programs. Job retraining for laid off employees is a variation of this concept.

Given the short-term severance and outplacement costs of work-force reductions, the savings in salaries are often overstated, particularly if cuts are not assumed to be the only way of eliminating poor performers. If one adds the costs of lower productivity and commitment, a case can be made for reducing the work force through attrition in conjunction with training and lateral or downward mobility. The attrition alternative is not sufficiently considered, because a cost-benefit analysis is rarely conducted. In times of adversity, finance and control functions, with their relatively short-term focus on quarterly earnings, gain power at the expense of the human resource function which takes a long-term perspective.

If an effective outplacement process allows separation without severe psychological or economic trauma, then why not induce employees to reexamine their places in the firm periodically instead of waiting for an economic downswing to force re-examination? This is the approach taken at Corning Glass Works. Every five years, bosses and personnel development specialists conduct reviews to determine whether it makes sense for an individual to remain with the firm given his or her needs, available opportunities, and the firm's view of his or her potential. A joint decision to stay or leave is agreed upon. Since both parties are presumably committed to the decision, separation, if it occurs, is less painful and more amicable. The firm's reputation in its labor markets is not damaged and it can go on to provide opportunities for other employees.

Tp sum up, policies affecting personnel outflow need to be considered as part of an organisation's overall strategy, since they will have a major impact on the commitment of employees and on the ability of the firm to be competitive. A combination of the policies and practices outlined above may make it possible for firms in the United States, where legislation has not yet restricted managerial freedom with respect to layoffs and termination, to find a path that balances employees' needs for reasonable employment security with the corporate need to maintain a quality and quantity of personnel consistent with being competitive.

Every society must deal with the problem of justice. Unless citizens believe they are treated fairly and have the opportunity for their grievances to be adjudicated, they will not be committed to that society; conflict and disintegration will result. Corporations as mini-societies are not exempt from the need to deal with the problem of fairness, particularly with respect to managing personnel flow. There are few issues on which employees or prospective employees feel more strongly than unfair practices with respect to hiring, promotion, and termination. The perception of the fairness of these policies is thus as strategically important to the organisation as the particular system and procedures selected to implement the policies. For that reason, we suggest that general managers, as well as staff specialists, need to give careful consideration to the fairness of their human resource flow policies.

Why is there such a decline in employee perception of fairness? It is quite likely that company practices have not gotten worse; indeed, they may even have improved. With the passing of equal opportunity legislation and greater emphasis in society on the rights of member ship, employees are more sensitised to their basic rights and more willing to articulate them. The ever increasing number of legal suits being brought against companies with regard to hiring, promotion, and termination supports this and makes it quite evident that management cannot ignore the fairness issue.

The Legal Perspective

In the United States, employers must comply with two major sets of regulations governing equal employment practices: Executive Order 11246 (as amended) and Title VII of the Civil Rights Act of 1964 (as amended). These provisions establish criteria by which discrimination is judged, notably comparing the selection ratios of minorities or women with those of whites or males and comparing numbers of minorities and women in the work force with their representation in the population of the community. Thus, intent to discriminate does not necessarily have to be proven (although recent Supreme Court rulings have made proof of intent a more important factor). In many other instances, the government can require employers to develop affirmative action programs (AAPs) aimed at redressing imbalances. It is not our intent to go into the details of these laws or the means by which the government enforces them.

Due Process Mechanisms

It is our intent to emphasise the importance of equal employment opportunity laws and regulations in the United States and to point to the consequences of their existence and of noncompliance with them. These laws represent a new standard by which employees and the community can judge a corporation. If management calls itself an equal opportunity employer, employees will feel more unjustly treated if they perceive discrepancies in actual practice than if management had not made such a claim. Under these circumstances, employees will feel much more strongly that changes must be made, and they will feel empowered to confront management directly, knowing they have legal recourse if no action is taken.

Management must create a mechanism for determining if complaints are valid and for resolving the problems if they are. This calls for an industrial jurisprudence, a process management can create for resolving grievances before grievances get to a court of law. David Ewing, who has studied how companies handle disputes, found few have appropriate means through which nonunion employees can voice a complaint or file a grievance. There are several types of complaint resolution processes that seem to work in the few companies that have them. Control Data and Polaroid use panels of managers and/or employees, who hear both sides of the case and decide what correction if any must be made.

Management Enforcement

There is little doubt that fair treatment of employees cannot spring from legal constraints alone, though these have provided the pressure for change in standards of fairness. Nor can fairness be obtained by the written policies of top management that have followed legislative pressures. Only the sincere belief of management in certain standards of fairness for all can result in a persistent top-down effort to enforce the standards and thereby change the values of managers throughout the corporation. The following strategies have to be employed in concert to achieve the needed changes in attitudes and behaviour throughout the corporation.

1. *The setting of clear goals* for hiring and promoting women, minorities, and other underutilised groups. Achievement of the goals must be rewarded and nonachievement must have negative consequences. Experience suggests that only companies that have such goals have had some success in enforcing standards of fairness.
2. *Clear articulation of top management values and philosophy* on fairness issues. What is meant by fairness? In particular, what constitutes a fair process?
3. *The development of due process systems* for resolving

complaints about hiring, performance evaluation, promotion, and termination decisions. The more power employees or their representatives are given to help adjudicate disputes, the more likely it is that change will occur and that perceptions of fairness will result.

4. *The creation of corporate policies and systems* that encourage fairness. These might include information systems to track the number of women and minorities who were hired, promoted, terminated, and who left voluntarily. They might also include performance appraisal and bonus systems that incorporate fairness considerations.
5. *Training and development* for managers and supervisors aimed at helping them understand the characteristics of a fair process and developing their skills in managing fairly a number of critical processes, including selection interviews and decisions about performance appraisal, pay, promotion, and termination.
6. *Awareness training* for employees, particularly women and minorities, which helps them clarify and articulate their career goals and teaches them how to utilise due-process mechanisms.

Ignoring or suppressing different views or disputes will have a negative impact, leading inevitably to dissatisfaction, turnover, low commitment, a poor-public image, and lawsuits. If feelings of unfair treatment are widespread in a democratic society, they will result in legislation that further reduces managerial freedom and flexibility.

Strategic Management of Flow

There are many systems and practices to manage the flow of human resources. The personnel function plays a central role in designing and administering many of the practices, but general managers are the only ones who can be responsible for articulating the philosophy that must guide the design and administration of these systems. Without such an articulation, human resource flow practices will not be internally consistent, nor will they support the firm's strategy or culture.

It is a general manager's responsibility to take a leadership role in deciding on a flow pattern and designing policies and systems that take these three areas into account. It is in this sense that we refer to human resource flow as a policy area. The process of continually discussing and monitoring who is being hired, transferred, promoted, terminated, or retired and the way these decisions fit the needs of the individual and the organisation are also responsibilities of the general manager.

Alternative Flow Patterns

There are three basic types of human resource flow patterns that may exist in an organisation, and a fourth type that is a mix of the first three.

1. *Lifelong employment system.* People usually enter the organisation at the bottom and stay with the organisation throughout their careers. The bottom may be defined differently for different employee groups. Blue-collar employees enter at the lowest job classification in the company, while MBAs are hired for entry-level exempt positions. No one is laid off as a result of economic cycles, but people may be asked to leave because of poor performance, depending on the company and on national practices. Large companies in Japan operate under this system. A select group of their employees are not discharged because of poor performance; instead, they may be sidetracked to less important jobs. Hewlett-Packard, IBM, and some other high-technology companies have a lifelong employment system, but poor performers can be terminated on a case-by-case

basis. In Europe, companies are forced to operate under this type of system because legislation makes the costs of termination prohibitive, particularly for older employees.

2. *Up-or-out system.* Employees enter at the bottom and move up through the organisation through predetermined tracks until they reach the top rank, which offers full partnership in the organisation and usually tenure. Inability to be promoted through any of the ranks along the way or to the highest rank usually means that the person must leave. This system has high levels of turnover at the bottom and relative stability at the top. Big Eight accounting firms, law firms, some management consulting firms, and university faculties are examples.

3. *Unstable in-and-out system.* Employees enter at any level in the organisation, depending on the organisation's need, and may be asked to leave at any level or point in their career because of economic conditions, poor performance, or lack of fit with new management. Sometimes, employment contracts exist for given periods to ensure individuals some stability. While this type of system is not restricted to any industry, it tends to be found in industries where performance is thought to be a function of the individual (rather than the group) and is highly variable (often due to factors outside the control of the individual). The entertainment industry (sports teams and network television) and many retailing organisations are examples. In-and-out patterns are found in the blue-collar work force where poor economic conditions trigger layoffs and good economic conditions result in hiring.

4. *Mixed patterns.* There are few corporations that are clearcut examples of one of the above. Large Japanese

companies have lifelong employment for their core employees while using an in-and-out system for temporary workers and women. Some companies operate a lifelong employment system for top management, but an in-and-out system for middle and lower management. Furthermore, flow patterns shift over the life cycle of an organisation.

In most cases, the choice of patterns selected by an organisation is less reflective of a coherent set of management attitudes and values than it is of the economic environment in which that organisation operates. If demand for a company's products is subject to severe economic fluctuations, the company is more likely to adopt an in-and-out flow pattern, subjecting employees to layoffs when poor economic conditions prevail.

On the other hand, a company in a rapidly growing industry may adopt a lifelong employment policy simply because it has never had to face severe economic decline. If the labor market has a large supply of needed talent, in-and-out flow patterns develop since they allow the firm to replace employees relatively easily. Choices about flow patterns also reflect societal values which can be imposed through legislation restricting the freedom of managers to terminate. Finally, flow patterns may be shaped by the philosophy of a corporation's founders.

Strategic Implications

Over time, a human resource flow pattern is institutionalised. Managers who know they will be asked to reduce employees at some point may be more careless about who they hire and how tightly they control headcount. They may purposely build a reserve of excess employees as a buffer against eventual cuts; this decision, in turn, makes reductions inevitable. The problem with this process is that it does not take into account the effects that institutionalised flow patterns have on the relationship between the organisation and its employees or the relationship of the corporation to society. A more strategic approach to human resource flow patterns would suggest that an organisation's general manager, supported by the expertise of his or her human resource staff, should weigh carefully the impact of such choices on a broad spectrum of key strategic outcomes, including employee commitment and competence, organisational adaptation and culture, the impact on interdependence and cooperation, and the relationship between the organisation and its host society.

Effects on employee competence. The flow pattern of an organisation affects how its managers think about the general task of managing. An in-and-out system fosters an emphasis on *selection* as opposed to *development*. If there are no constraints or identifiable costs to hiring and firing, why invest efforts in developing employees? On the other hand, if firing employees is difficult or costly, managers will become more careful in selection and will invest more in development. That developmental approach may increase the competence of employees as well as change the relationship between the organisation and the employee. Employees who believe they are receiving an opportunity for development often feel a greater sense of commitment to the organisation.

Effects on employee commitment. Employees who know that terminations or layoffs may come any time the economy takes a downturn will think differently about their relationship to the organisation than employees who know they have a job until retirement. Insecure employees are likely to be more calculating about the relationship, deciding to stay only so long as their career needs are met quickly. Employees who expect to be with the company until retirement are likely to take a longer-term view of their relationship to the organisation. They may be willing to accept slower promotions or temporary setbacks in their career aspirations without lowering commitment. Up-and-out firms may be successful in obtaining high levels of motivation from younger employees who seek promotion, but are likely to incur problems of motivation or "burnout" among senior employees. Thus, different flow patterns and the policies about employment security, advancement, or demotion that shape them cause employees to develop different rationalisations for why they are working and why they are working for a particular company. Are they working to accumulate rewards such as money and promotion that they can take with them to another company or are they working to contribute to an institution from which they will retire? Different flow patterns create quite different "psychological contracts" between the individual and the organisation.

We are saying that some flow patterns (notably in-and-out and up-or-out patterns) make it difficult for employees to develop long-term commitment to an organisation, even when other factors such as satisfaction with work, pay, and working conditions may make commitment desirable. Thus, some flow patterns may make it more difficult for managers to develop commitment and competence in employees. Lifelong employment creates a base for building commitment and competence, assuming management can develop effective policies in the areas of employee influence, rewards, and work systems.

Effects on organisational adaptation. Flow patterns may also affect the organisation's adaptive capacities. Some American managers argue that periodic work-force reductions force managers to weed out dead wood, and provide opportunities to reshape the organisation with a new breed of employees. This is one method for managing change. The argument suggests that organisations with in-and-out flow patterns are likely to have more diversity among employees. It is generally accepted that diversity contributes to innovation. Newcomers, not yet socialised by the organisation, see old problems in new ways and propose different solutions. It is widely speculated that Japanese companies may not be as innovative as American companies, because of their lifetime employment system. Diversity can, however, be built into firms with lifetime employment if they systematically recruit people with different backgrounds and traits. On the other hand, in-and-out and up-or-out systems are likely to experience problems with adaptation because new people moving rapidly through lower levels do not have the power or network of relationships to create major changes or cannot afford to take risks.

Effects on interdependence. Cooperation in organisations may occur because formal structures direct people to work interdependently. Matrix structures, task forces, special coordinating roles, and reward systems can be used to encourage collaboration between interdependent groups and individuals. But interpersonal relationships can be a more powerful means than formal structures for encouraging cooperation. Senior employees in lifetime employment systems and partners in up-or-out systems develop a network of relationships that make it easier to coordinate interdependent parts of the organisation. In Japanese companies cooperation is achieved in the absence of many formal structures because their lifetime employment system allows relationships to develop.

Effects on culture. Each organisation has its own cultures, a set of shared beliefs and values that guide employee behavior. However, organisations differ in the strength of their corporate cultures. Culture is so pervasive in some organisations that it is an extremely powerful force in shaping behavior, while in other organisations values are not as widely shared and have less of an impact on employee behavior. Strong cultures develop more easily in lifetime systems because employees are more likely to identify with the organisation and want to become socialised. Furthermore, a stable pool of senior employees can help with the socialisation of new members. An up-or-out system can also develop a strong culture, but the burden of maintaining the culture falls on a relatively small number of senior employees. Managers of high-commitment work systems who want to use culture as a means of social control and want to develop a clan-like organisation will have to consider these factors in choosing a human resource flow pattern.

Flow patterns can also influence *the type of culture* that an organisation develops, particularly with respect to how power is distributed.

In-and-out flow patterns reflect different assumptions about the role of the corporation in society than do lifetime employment systems. The former assumes that employees exist for the purpose of helping the corporation make a profit. The latter assumes that the corporation exists to provide stable employment and a meaningful existence for workers. These assumptions are usually implicit. Only occasionally do managers explicitly ask what the purpose of the corporation in society is. Are profits an end or a means to some other end? Lifetime employment fits that concept. Similarly, European legislation regarding the termination rights of employees reflects the implicit belief of those societies that the purpose of the corporation is to provide employment and that profit is not an end, but a means. American managers, on the other hand, usually operate under the assumption that profits are the primary goal of the corporation.

The discussion above suggests that human resource flow patterns can affect employer-employee relationships in several important ways, just as they reflect management's implicit assumptions about the purpose of the corporation. However, in many corporations, flow patterns are shaped in a reactive way by the situational forces in the history of the company. This suggests that general managers would be well advised to examine their human resource flow pattern, the rationale underlying it, and its consequences for some of the variables we have discussed.

A strategic decision to change the flow pattern might then follow, and that decision could contribute significantly to reshaping all four HRM outcomes: commitment, competence, congruence, and cost effectiveness. Examination of flow patterns could lead to policy innovations that combine the advantages of both lifetime employment and in-and-out systems and nullify the disadvantages of both. For example, if lifetime employment provides a sense of security for employees but could lead to an obsolescent work force and high costs in a recessionary economy, might it not be possible to obtain both psychological security and the flexibility that management seeks by providing *career*, not *job* security.

Flow Policies/Systems Designing

The choice of a flow pattern will probably emerge from a careful examination and discussion of many of the policies and issues discussed in this chapter. When and how should recruiting be done? How should employee effectiveness be defined and evaluated? How should this information be used in personnel decisions and career development? What systems and practices should the company adopt for developing employees, and what philosophy should guide this process?

These are questions that should be answered explicitly by general managers with the help of key managers and human resource specialists. When a system for examining and shaping flow patterns is lacking, an organisation's history and its immediate problems will shape these patterns in ways that may not fit the company's strategic needs.

A top management group should take time periodically to examine the type of information described above to answer the questions suggested. Some companies have commissioned audits by outside consultants. The consultants collect information by examining records and conducting interviews, then report to top management. Some of the data can be supplied by the human resource function, particularly by a competent personnel research department. With this type of information in hand, top management and key line managers should engage in a dialogue to clarify for themselves corporate strategy and philosophy. In the final analysis, flow policies reflect the assumptions of top management about human competence and development in the context of business reality.

Planning Human Resource Flow

How would you determine numbers and types of employees? How would you determine who stays and who goes? The answers to these questions can only emerge from a flow planning process, which may be formal or informal, quantitative or judgmental, long- or short-term. The plan may be aimed at assuring a supply of employees in all categories (i.e., engineers, production personnel, secretaries, managers), or it may be aimed at only one or two critical groups such as engineers and managers. Finally, the planning process may encompass the entire company or just a smaller group of key executives and technical personnel. Regardless of the focus, the process encompasses the same basic steps.

1. *Forecast* the number and types of employees that will be needed (labor demand) and the number and types of employees that will be available in the organisation (labor supply) assuming certain rates of turnover, transfers, and promotions.
2. *Program* recruiting, employee development, and/or outplacement to deal with anticipated shortages and surpluses.

3. *Evaluate* the effectiveness of personnel programs in dealing with surpluses and shortages, and revise the plan where necessary.

A quantitative forecast of demand can be made by using certain leading indicators that have a demonstrated relationship to personnel requirements. The problem with this approach is that it assumes the future to be an extrapolation of the past, an unwarranted assumption in a rapidly changing environment. Alternatively, management can try to project the implications of changes in markets, technology, and strategy for the structure of the organisation and the strength and size of certain functions and roles. From this, a forecast of personnel needs can be developed, particularly one that highlights changes in requirements. Management groups that engage in this qualitative forecasting process often find many side benefits such as a clarification of strategy, changing functional roles and relationships, and emerging structural arrangements. The demand forecasting process can lead management to address difficult organisational issues before serious problems develop. Effective demand forecasting requires a blend of quantitative and qualitative approaches, using each to check and inform the other. While the procedure for forecasting supply is well established, the effectiveness of the procedure depends heavily on good personnel data. Even when performance evaluation data are obtained, managers may not always report accurately their assessments of subordinates or their intentions to fire or promote if they don't know how this data will be used. Nor do companies know exactly who is planning to quit. Through an examination of historical patterns, some estimates may be made but these are highly problematical. This is why *aggregated forecasting,* which projects supply for a group of employees using sophisticated models, does not usually yield very useful information, though it may be of some value as a check on a *disaggregated approach to forecasting supply.*

This approach, commonly referred to as succession or replacement planning, relies on the personal knowledge of managers to estimate who might quit or retire and who should be promoted or terminated. In replacement planning, managers are asked to designate individuals whom they regard as *backups* for their or other key jobs. Individuals are chosen on the basis of their experience and evaluation of performance and potential. By comparing demand estimates and supply estimates, a shortage or surplus may be identified for each category of employee within the company to which the process is applied. Action plans are then devised by line managers to deal with filling gaps or terminating employees. The critical link in the flow planning process is *follow-up*.

Even after managers have established procedures, development programs do not always follow. If individuals who were to receive specific training or job experiences do not, the company will find itself lacking the needed technical and managerial talent. These are "soft" programs that are difficult to define, preprogram, and measure. Increasingly, corporations are finding that flow planning needs to be tied to the strategic planning process. These corporations will not accept a business plan from a manager unless it provides a flow analysis. When these plans are reviewed periodically and managers are rewarded for their accomplishment, they are more likely to be implemented. If the corporation wishes to reward managers who successfully develop people, it is important that follow-up include not only a monitoring of activities (training programs, recruitment programs, etc.) but also developmental results (the number of successful technical or managerial personnel promoted from a unit).

Besides its analytic nature, succession planning is also a *subjective process*. Employees who are candidates for promotion in the in the eyes of one manager may be viewed negatively by other managers applying different standards. In any case, succession in a corporation must be agreed to by a number of key managers, all of whom will have to work with the person in question. For this reason many companies have developed a committee process for reviewing key managerial personnel at every level of the organisation.

Conclusion

Managing the flow of people *in, through,* and *out* of the corporation is a human resource policy area of strategic importance to corporations. Policy decisions in this area require that general managers adopt more than just an enterprise perspective. They must also understand the perspective of the individual, particularly in regard to what constitutes career development and satisfaction. Additionally, they must develop a societal perspective, which involves an understanding of changing worker values, educational institutions that supply prospective recruits, legislation, government regulatory agencies, and union policy. To assure the right numbers of employees with a mix of skills required to implement corporate strategy, corporations must design appropriate policies and practices for managing employee inflow, internal flow, and outflow. A number of important questions and issues must be addressed to develop effective flow policies. How can employees be recruited that will fit the organisation's needs and culture? What is the optimum velocity of personnel flow through the corporation consistent with good employee development and the strategic needs of the organisation? How is employee effectiveness defined and how shall it be evaluated? How can an organisational context be created that will encourage employee development? What mechanisms and processes can corporations install to meet employee expectations for fairness in connection with hiring, promotion, and termination decisions? Finally, should the company terminate, retire early, or otherwise encourage employees to leave when profits drop? What alternatives exist to this policy?

The four types of patterns are identified: lifelong employment, up-or-out, in-and-out, and a mixed pattern of all three types. Each has a quite different impact on important outcomes such as commitment, competence, and organisational culture and adaptibility.

General managers must make strategic choices about the flow pattern they want and the policies and practices that will be needed to support their choice. Such strategic choices will be a function of competitive realities, stakeholder interests, and management's values with regard to employee development and security. A continuous process of examining values, the effects of current flow policies, and the future goals of the firm will allow managers to shape flow patterns and policies. One ongoing responsibility of general managers is to be involved in planning and managing personnel flow within the context of existing policies.

How many managers, professionals, specialists, or skilled workers will the firm require to meet its business goals? What mix of recruiting and employee development programs will be needed to serve those needs? Who are the managers and professionals with the highest potential to succeed incumbents in key positions? These are questions that should be addressed as part of the business planning process. Many modern organisations create special forums where key managers at each level of the organisation discuss key people, their potential, and their developmental needs.

9

MANAGING HUMAN RESOURCES IN PRACTICE

> "Many imagine that the higher you go, the easier the climbing. Don't be governed by that theory unless you have a soft place to fall back into."
>
> —*J.L. Boggus*

At the very least, it would seem that there is an evident commonality of language and ideas permeating employing organizations in diverse sectors. Managers in health care, motor vehicle assembly, railways, brewing and local government are busy with talk of 'visioning', of clarifying organizational 'mission', of promoting 'managerial leadership' and pursuing 'excellence' through, among other devices, effective communication, the linking of reward with performance, more systematic selection and through a more 'committed' and 'adaptable' workforce. Only a few years ago most of these managers would not have been using this language and probably would not even have heard of some of these terms. But is it only the language which has changed or is there evidence to suggest that something more fundamental is happening in the way that employees are managed?

The 27 dimensions are condensed by homing-in on the HRM variant. The scoring methodology is inevitably rather simplistic; it is indicative rather than definitive. A tick is allocated to a cell when the particular HRM-type characteristic was found to be broadly in evidence or where there were signs that significant energy was being expended to bring this state of affairs into being that is it was a significant agenda item for certain key managerial players. A cross is allocated when none of the above conditions applied to any marked degree and a question mark is shown where either the item was on the agenda, though not a pressing issue, or where certain parts of the organization such as a particular division or business unit had registered the dimension as a key agenda item.

The patterns on the figure can be regarded as a pictorial representation of the welter of initiatives being taken by managements at this time. Of course, what the figure cannot do is reveal any of the subtle aspects associated with these moves. These aspects will require exploration across a number of chapters. In this present chapter the task is begun by examining, in turn, each of the main component spheres of human resource management. This is done in three sections: the first examines initiatives associated with the resourcing and utilizing of labour; the second section focuses on changes in leadership and motivation; the third and final section attends to training and developmental practices.

RESOURCING AND UTILIZATION

Under this heading we will review developments in the practices of:

- human resource planning
- deployment and utilization
- recruitment and selection

Human Resource Planning

It may have been a response to the demographic message and to the already tight labour markets in certain parts of the country in the late 1980s, but whatever the reason, there were signs that more attention was being paid to human resource planning.

Notoriously, the HR planning process has been the arena for prescription with a dearth of hard, evidence that practice was in any way being affected. Even today, despite recent uncertainties about the state of labour supply, there is no reliable source of information about the extent to which companies do take a strategic approach to the acquisition, retention, utilization and improvement of their human resources. Surveys by NEDO (1988, 1989) and others, suggested that significant numbers of employers had an inadequate understanding of the demographic profiles of the workforce in the 1990s and it seems that even among those employers who did appreciate these changes, few had formulated plans for responding to the situation. One could begin to suggest that outside the traditional lifetime employment organizations, such as the large clearing banks or the civil service, many, if not most, employers continue with an essentially *ad hoc* and pragmatic approach to their human resourcing problems.

To a large extent, the findings from the 15 large case studies reported here would tend to support this suspicion. Even the basic raw data about the employed population in these organizations frequently did not exist in a usable form for planning purposes. For example, in the National Health Service, the way in which central statistics were collected meant that the Regional and District Health Authorities did not have a composite picture of the number of different types of nurses available. In effect, psychiatric nurses were being counted in with nurses who had specialized in paediatrics, and theatre-nurse statistics were computed alongside general ward nurses. Similarly, in the private sector engineering companies, human resource planning was also found to be frequently rudimentary. Even senior management succession planning, for instance, was in the main left to informal and *ad hoc* mechanisms devised by particular individuals. And even among the more sophisticated cases, where central personnel had drawn up a standardized mechanism complete with formal succession plans and elaborate profiles of the managerial stock, it was often admitted that the resultant piles of forms were hardly used because the information was quickly outdated.

Such instances might be considered particularly surprising given the number of commercial software packages on the market which purport to offer computerized human resource planning. Over half of the cases in our sample had in fact subscribed to one of these services but, typically, they were in the early stages of adapting them for planning purposes as opposed to the long standing practice of using them for simple personnel records. One of the main difficulties was that while these systems purportedly allowed for inclusion of training records, experience and capabilities on the databases, the information stored was usually considered too schematic to be really useful for planning purposes. Typically, it was said that a trawl through such files might be undertaken in order to construct a 'long list' of possibles when moves were being planned, but, that the fine judgements required individual sifting. Even the suppliers of these planning systems were found not to be using them in their own organizations. Part of the reluctance to pin too much hope at this time on computerized human resource planning stems from the backlash to a premature attempt to produce 'mechanistic' planning systems in the 1970s. These were considered to be abstract and intricate mathematical exercises which served to produce technical models of supply and demand but which seemed to have little practical use. Put simply, the forecasts were frequently inaccurate and the implications for action were not clear.

But it would be wrong to conclude from this that no strategic thinking about resourcing was occurring in these organizations at the time of the study. One of the clearest examples was in fact found among the wider 'panel' of cases. Golden Wonder employs 3000 people on six sites. After the Hanson Trust takeover of the company from the Imperial Group, the company trod water for a while before being sold to Dalgety. The industrial relations approach of Golden Wonder has traditionally rested on company level bargaining for most of the process operators. The pattern of relations in the various functions was described within the company as non-participative and even 'authoritarian'. But, on the human resource planning front, the company has taken a coordinated series of initiatives. The workload in crisp manufacture fluctuates depending upon seasonal peaks and special sales promotions. A temporary workers' agreement caters for employees engaged for periods up to 26 weeks. In any one factory the number of temporaries can range from zero to as many as 500. An average, however, would be some 200 temporaries for a few peak months.

There is 24-hour, three-shift working. In 1985 a proposal was put to the unions suggesting three categories of employees. Category One was to be the permanent workforce; Category Two would be permanent part-timers that is those working two to three days per week but with an 'agreed flexibility' to work the extra two or three days in the week (for which no overtime would be paid until 39 hours was reached). A third Category was to be composed of the temporary staff. A ballot of the workforce led, however, to rejection of this scheme.

With the help of a team of management consultants the company then turned to what was known as an 'annual hours' package which involved the averaging out of total hours worked over a 12-month period so that what was worked in any particular week was no longer regarded as the critical factor. It entoiled a planned reduction in work hours for the first category and an increase for the other two categories. The planning of the annual hours and the mixed composition of the labour force to reach the total required was accompanied by an 'integrated approach'. A policy document was produced which linked the issues of harmonization of conditions, training, progression, rewards and the flexible use of the different categories of labour. The company also seriously considered 'no-strike agreements' and to this end, managers visited various Japanese sites in Britain in order to glean ideas. The TGWU was seen as an obstacle to aspirations of this sort, however. The company has a personnel director sitting on the board and human resource planning issues of the kind indicated, feature regularly in board discussions. There was a strike-which affected most parts of the company in 1985 but since that date the integrated package has been rolled-out in a very determined way. In formal terms the 15 case companies might easily claim to undertake human resource planning if prompted to reply to a survey question. But in practice, its usage was found to be very limited. Hence, this first tenet of the HRM model was found wanting.

Deployment and Utilization

A conscious attempt to construct an integrated approach to human resource planning and utilization is also strongly in evidence at another food-processing company: Birds Eye Walls. Birds Eye is the frozen food subsidiary of the Anglo-Dutch Unilever company. The planning here centres on an attempt to alter radically the assumptions about the nature of labour requirements. The central thrust hinges on a plan to introduce 'teamworking'. This entails fully interchangeable process teams so that each individual can not only do other people's process-related jobs but, in addition, the teams are also responsible for their own routine maintenance. On a day-to-day basis each team decides who will do which task, including information inputting on shopfloor keyboards.

The team-focused human resource planning is part of a wider initiative across the Birds Eye Walls company known as 'Workstyle'. This package was carefully planned and negotiated in a series of working groups with employee representatives from each area. Agreement was reached with these groups, which included shop steward representatives, on measures which amounted to near total flexibility. This lengthy consultative negotiation process was undertaken on a site-by-site basis: failure to reach agreement at the Kirkby location was one of the reasons for the closure of that facility. The level of flexibility and associated training across specialized tasks was apparently more than met overall. One manager suggested that they had actually got more than was needed:

> We got it wrong: we have found we don't actually need mat level of interchangeability. For a team of 10 to be efficient you may need only 7 to be able to do *x* and, say, 6 to be able to do *y*. We initially went for the whole lot. This, we later found was not necessary.

While the process operators teams were found to be fully operable, the engineers and electricians had drawn back. The aim was to combine fitters and electricians in 'mechanical-electrical/electronic teams'. Their fears were countered by managers who said, 'Don't worry about past job boundaries. Focus on the new sophisticated equipment we are introducing; that's what we want you to be concerned about'.

But the integrated planning process extends beyond team-working and flexibility. A number of erstwhile full-time employees have been switched onto part-time working. The Grimsby plant, for example, gained a majority of employees voting for this move as a means of 'saving the factory'. The resultant part-time resourced, four-shift pattern is highly economical with curtailed overtime, no shift payments and reduced holiday entitlement.

There is no doubting the way in which human resource planning has contributed a crucial element in the business plan. 'Workstyle' is billed within the company as an HRM initiative designed to underpin the rationalization programme, part of which is the concentration of production of frozen foods into a few technologically-sophisticated sites. As part of this the distribution side has been sold off to National Freight.

The factory closures and the simultaneous investment in new technology in the remaining sites were seen to open up an ideal opportunity to introduce a 'people-management change programme'. The plan was an attempt to 'harness initiative' the stated aim was to raise expectations and to tap into that decision-making capability which, ordinary workers display in their work lives outside working hours.

The 'Workstyle' initiative was described as 'holistic': it was frequently drawn in diagram form comprising the three interrelated pillars of: 'responsibility/flexibility/quality'. The attainment of these three constituent features was seen to depend upon the teamworking concept The package was presented as a means to make work more interesting and to foster greater responsibility. For example, Workstyle is described by the company thus:

Workstyle which was introduced at Gloucester and

> Lowestoft is a concept which gives employee workgroups the responsibility for organising their own work, by their own methods, leaving management free to manage. Workgroup members are encouraged to understand every aspect of the production process from start to finish and to take responsibility for meeting quality, cost and tonnage targets.
>
> (Birds Eye Walls Annual Report and Accounts, 1986)

As part of this concept, supervision was removed and the teams became self-supervising. In practice, however, the shift managers, to a large extent, still behaved as if they were doing the supervisory job. The managers were supposed to be raising their sights so as to tackle wider issues such as identifying training needs, setting priorities, auditing team performance, health and safety, planning and advising the production managers. Each shift manager (assistant manager) was typically responsible for two teams of 10 persons. They were held to account, in the final analysis, for the actions of these groups. As senior managers saw it: 'We have to have a single person we can go to carry the responsibility'. In consequence, some assistant managers responded by being 'too interventionary' that is behaving as if they were still supervisors. Others 'back-off too far and control has slipped'.

Taken together, the two cases of Golden Wonder and Birds Eye indicate that there are examples of consciously planned and, indeed, strategic action with regard to the resourcing and utilization of the workforce. The mechanistic manpower-planning models have been superseded and there is clearly evidence of a type of planning which attends not only to regulating numbers but is proactive in respect of part-time work and annual hours contracts, and proactive in the realm of radically different forms of labour utilization.

This latter is illustrated particularly with the teamworking initiatives at Birds Eye which was dissolving traditional job boundaries and even helping to remove the whole supervisory tier.

Nonetheless, the two cases along with the other examples cited, also point to the difficulties which these sorts of initiatives encounter. Removing supervision leads some managers to try to fill that role themselves; it leads others virtually to abandon work teams to their own devices. The Workstyle agreements at Birds Eye have yet to embrace the critical constituency of maintenance workers. And at Golden Wonder, the new working patterns remain subject to future negotiation with the trade unions and cannot therefore be regarded as installed in perpetuity.

A key aspect of labour utilization in the 1980s was of course the question of the flexible deployment of the available labour resource. The concept of 'flexibility' loomed large in debate. Indeed, it figured so prominently that it sometimes appeared that this intermediate objective represented what many managerial change programmes have been largely about. Against the back-cloth of controversy on this theme, what contribution can be made by the findings from these detailed case studies?

The first point to note was that, overall, the efforts spent by management to secure flexibility across a whole number of fronts was found to be considerable. Initiatives designed to achieve more flexibility in labour utilization were particularly notable in the manufacturing companies. For example, Plessey Naval Systems signed a formal 'Flexibility Agreement' with the EETPU. This stated that:

(i) existing hourly paid demarcation practices be replaced by total flexibility

(ii) the definition of 'total flexibility' is that employees will carry out every task within their capability

(iii) to achieve flexible manning it will be necessary for employees to learn new skills and develop existing skills

(iv) deployment will be based on business needs

(v) a revised flexibility grading structure will be introduced.

Four grades were introduced based on experience and capability. Ironically, as the bulk of the work was becoming more standardized and de-skilled the implied necessity for skill enhancement proved to be somewhat illusory. The expansion largely occurred in the lowest grade and even some apprenticed trained skilled workers able, for example, to work from drawings, found themselves spending more of their days on routine assembly.

With the introduction of microelectronics into the Coventry telecommunications site of GEC, (another of our 'panel' companies), a similar situation was found to be developing. The implication that can be drawn from this is that strategic choice with regard to flexible utilization of labour will be influenced by technology. The drive for functional flexibility was, in general, especially important in manufacturing, but its importance varied considerably between situations where de-skilled operatives rendered it superfluous to those semi-skilled areas where the lack of interchange between tasks was seen as a major obstacle to be overcome. This latter situation prevailed most noticeably in the motor companies. At Ford, Jaguar, Peugeot and Austin Rover, there were definite attempts to facilitate inter-craft working and to expand the jobs of semi-skilled operatives to take in maintenance, inspection, cleaning and some responsibility for ensuring a smooth supply of material to the work stations. In British

Rail, a key initiative has been the 'traincrew concept' which has breached the long-standing divide between drivers and guards. The 1988 Traincrew Agreement reached between BR, the NUR and ASLEF provided for a new grade structure which is described as 'fully versatile':

> The occupant of the post whether designated Train (wo)man (Driver) or Train (wo)man (Guard) will perform the duties of the other grade provided training in that role has been received.
>
> (1988 Traincrew Agreement, Clause 5)

Measures of this kind are of course not entirely new: productivity bargaining in the 1960s as exemplified in Flanders' account of the *Fawley Blue Book* (1964) illustrates the point. But what is different is the extensiveness of the changes and the way in which they are underpinned by related developments. Thus, for example, a common observation in the 1960s and 1970s was that the buy-out of 'restrictive practices' was often phoney: in part because the agreements were frequently a thinly disguised side-stepping of the statutory incomes policies and in part because modified 'restrictions' emerged in their place. Under the current climate the accompanying real and extensive reductions in headcounts (as much as 30-40 per cent has been common in the larger manufacturing concerns) have meant that the pressure on those remaining to change their job scope has been of an entirely different order than before. This is not to say that flexibility' is necessarily sought as an end in itself or that it is always and everywhere desired by management. Patently this is hot so. There are numerous instances where total flexibility is not seen as an appropriate goal. Management may expressly want a limited number of experienced workers to remain dedicated to a particular task swapping and changing around would be regarded as wasteful and even dangerous. Similarly, the costs of achieving flexibility whether incurred through training or through extra payment for skill attainment may also deter.

Ford Motor Company provides an excellent example of the various levels of complexity. In 1989 the announcement was made that Dagenham, on the assembly side, was to lose the 'contract' for the larger, prestige models and would be reduced to the assembly of the small car, the Fiesta. This widely publicized event was simply one further step in a longer-standing series of cross-cutting calculations which involves, on a European-wide canvas, relative productivity, changes to working practices, quality, and inter-plant competition.

In retrospect, the 1985 agreement for Ford of Britain was a turning point and it serves to illustrate the way in which the company intended to head in the future. This agreement contained a crucial element which made part of the deal contingent upon productivity gains. The novel aspect was that although Ford retained company-level national bargaining, the productivity allowances package was devolved to plant level for detailed attention. These discussions and the resulting agreements were both extensive. The broad principles are incorporated in the national agreement. This states: 'productivity allowances are payable to employees who cooperate with local management in ensuring maximum capacity utilization and the efficient use of manpower.' The 'changed work practices' are itemized based on the three 'principles of versatility and flexibility; the acquisition and use of new skills; the elimination of inefficient lines of demarcation'.

The agreement set out the requirements for production operators and for craft employees. Regarding the former, it is stated that in order to qualify for the productivity allowances, operators must, as required:

(i) seek, identify and repair defects (this includes the inspection and rectification of incoming work);

(ii) be involved in techniques, such as statistical process control, to record and use results from control process measures;

(iii) line feeding operators must procure and feed material to the work-place using the designated material handling equipment as required;

(iv) make adjustments to, clean and lubricate equipment this includes making corrections to settings, replacing worn parts and assisting, 'within their capability', craft employees who are carrying out maintenance duties.

As for craft employees, electrical and mechanical craftsmen 'must be flexible and versatile across the full range of their respective skills, and undertake any electrical or mechanical tasks outside their own trade subject to capabilities that are necessary to complete an assignment.' Both crafts have agreed to make the necessary preparations for work on equipment, including the use of lifting equipment and driving. They 'must also carry out line patrol, taking corrective actions as they identify the need and be mobile across a plant or operation' (The 1985 Agreement: 86).

While crossover between electrical and mechanical skills is not seen as attainable (for technical reasons) other than at the margins, the mechanical craftsmen 'must acquire and apply the full range of mechanical skills from all the mechanical trades' including advanced pneumatics and hydraulics. Payment is subject to meeting the standards set out in a formal training programme. The conditions specify that whether in body and assembly or powertrain, mechanical craftsmen are expected to be 'fully interchangeable' not only within their own traditional work areas 'but also central shop or toolroom and shopfloor maintenance'.

These conditions as set out in the national agreement are seen as the broad parameters: the detailed applications are the subject of local arrangement between plant management and 'in consultation with employees and their representatives'. As part of the deal the job evaluation system was abandoned and so too the grievance procedure for job grading.

So much for the formal agreement. But what has actually happened in the plants? The general estimate from various line managers at Dagenham and Halewood in 1987 was that they had, in fact, achieved 80 per cent of the conditions. Moreover, the remaining 20 per cent was usually seen as impeded by the want of investment in, for example, appropriate decentralized toolrooms (or 'cribs') rather than as a consequence of labour restriction. Allowance has to be made for a degree of bullishness in these crude estimates but even the stewards tended to endorse the general view that significant departures had been made from traditional practices, as a result of the agreements. A measure of reversion to past practice may, however, be expected. Already, for example, it was evident that where new dispersed 'cribs' for the mechanicals had been constructed in the machining and assembly areas, there was some struggle over the attempts by the craftsmen to develop these into closed havens instead of the envisaged open-plan workshops. Thus, attempts by the maintenance workers to have the cribs made fully enclosed with doors, ceilings and the like, were met with compromise agreements that resulted in the uppermost wall panels being sloped inwards so as to form semi-enclosed units. This small site of contention might be seen as likely to presage a more prolonged struggle over the amount of 'line patrolling' which can be expected.

Nevertheless, it would be a mistake to underestimate the degree of change. Underpinning the NJNC agreement on flexibility have been local plant agreements prompted by an entirely different calculation — namely, new work practices as a precondition for attracting investment in the face of inter-plant competition. This has been a feature of the engine plants in particular. Bridgend and Dagenham have had to compete for programmes for which continental plants, such as Cologne have been strong contenders. It has to be remembered that Ford is organized on a European basis for its manufacturing operations. The sourcing of any component, be it engine, gearbox, body or whatever, is thus potentially always a matter for inter-plant competition. The winning, in July 1985, of the in-line four-cylinder double-overhead camshaft engine for the Granada and Sierra models by Dagenham when it was initially regarded as destined for Cologne is a key case in point. To attract the £160m investment necessary to under-take this, Dagenham had to submit a detailed case built around changed working practices and cooperative labour relations. A series of off-site meetings between senior stewards and the plant management resulted in an extensive brochure documenting the agreed 'quantum change'. This involved locating skilled workers on production lines, oiling by operatives, mobility of labour within indirect functions and outsourcing of certain operations including some plant engineering.

In pursuit of these sorts of 'radical and far reaching' changes it is recognized that works committees are often placed in a difficult position *vis-a-vis* national officials and committees representing other locations. Accordingly, rather than insist on strict formal agreement, a 'tacit acceptance' was often deemed sufficient by plant managers. Conveners and senior stewards from the various plants tended to argue that while they face criticism from their colleagues for agreeing to major working practices' concessions, their critics were themselves 'hypocritically involved in similar agreements'.

There is also a considerable amount of exploration of

'scenarios'. In one plant during a joint meeting between senior management and senior stewards, the talk turned to future aspirations concerning the staffing of the machining area. The aim was clearly stated of having a 'team' of a dozen: four or five of whom would be oriented towards maintenance. Moreover, the production jobs were described as 'not old-fashioned production jobs' but ones entailing fault-tracing, monitoring, tool changing, adjusting and the like. It was estimated that such a team could itself take care of 75 per cent of the breakdowns which currently require the call-out of a maintenance engineer.

A twin-level push existed at Ford then. Locally, plants had to demonstrate cooperation and productivity (which is likely to involve, *inter alia*, flexible working) while at national level, the NJNC negotiated national agreement (the Blue Book) continued as an authoritative document which was amended from time to time. Also at national level, a Productivity Study Group had been meeting and this had buttressed the changes to working practices discussed above with a set of proposals relating to reform of the wage structure, which it identified as an inhibitor of flexible operation. As a result of this work, 500 job titles have been reduced to just 50. And, after 17 years of operation, the job evaluation process has been discarded in a move designed to allow line managers to be more directly responsible for the flexible use of the labour resource under their charge.

The overall view at Ford among the line managers charged with operating the system was a general satisfaction that at last the company had taken steps to improve productivity which had made a real and sustained impact. Indeed, the judgement seems to be that the company got far more out of the 1985 agreement than it had expected. The 1987 negotiations which led to a national strike were viewed, in contrast, as merely seeking the icing on the cake.

Peugeot-Talbot at Ryton in Coventry is another car manufacturer which has dramatically increased productivity. In the Peugeot case there is less room for doubt that the gains have resulted from cost cutting and new working practices rather than from investment in new advanced technology. Ryton remains a technologically traditional car plant given the present volume throughput (80,000 units per year). Nonetheless, productivity increased 100 per cent between 1980-8.

Here too, the changes to working practices have, in the main, resulted from a bargaining-for-change approach. In 1987 a new multi-craft grade (A+) with a 5 per cent differential was proposed. Until that time the manual grade classification had been 'A' to 'E' with grade 'A' being the highest. It contained, for example, toolmakers, electricians and pattern makers. Negotiations at Peugeot include the national officers of the main unions (TGWU, ASTMS, AEU, EETPU). Agreement and introduction were not finally achieved until 1990. To qualify for the new grade, the craftworker has to have passed a specified training programme and be doing work of the specified kind. Until the late 1980s, maintenance typically involved a number of different specialists for example, an electrician to isolate a defective machine, a millwright to remove the guard and undertake initial dismantling, and a toolmaker to repair the motor.

It is notable that Peugeot was not seeking full multi-trade working for all its craftworkers. It simply did not see the need for this, nor (and most important) did it want to pay for it. The limited amount of multi-craft working which the company sought was designed to involve what was described as the 'brighter of the toolmakers' receiving electrical and electronic training. After initial resistance, the stewards representing electricians have now shown a willingness to cooperate in this measure of multi-skilling.

The actual requirement for these multi-skilled. A+ grade' craftsmen was viewed as likely to vary across plants. Initial estimates were that 20 per cent of craftworkers would qualify for this grade at Ryton where only a few hightech machines were currently in place, but a much higher proportion at Stoke where the factory management seemed to want nearly all their skilled people to be fully flexible. (Up to 90 per cent was initially envisaged by plant managers.) Central personnel was seeking to reconcile these wide disparities.

Even before this 1987 move, some considerable flexibility was in evidence especially in the machine areas where operators were doing their own inspection, material collection, oiling and cleaning. These practices were coyly described as having simply 'evolved'.

In the main assembly areas the job-specifications remained more or less as they were. Few initiatives had been taken here where the prime requirement was routine and dependable accomplishment of fragmented tasks. The claimed outcome of attention to detail on the productivity chase is a regular schedule achievement rate of over 90 per cent Indeed 100 per cent was said to be attained quite often. Between 1983 and 1988 there was a productivity increase which saw Ryton come from 30 per cent behind the French plants to an equal position during a period when the French plants themselves have increased their own rate of productivity. Ryton moved, as a result, to double-shift working.

The body-in-white at Peugeot-Talbot illustrates the point about how reduced manning implies a combining of jobs and an expansion of responsibility. At the end of the body-in-white-line there used to be 12 metal finishers, 3 inspectors and 2 additional rectifiers. One area manager commented:

> The rectifiers saw it as part of their role to try to slip jobs past the inspectors. Now we have just 7

> men who do viewing and rectifying. Each is responsible for a particular car; they sign-off for it and they have a vested interest in it.

Notably, the manager continued by saying 'a problem is that they can be too good, that is be insufficiently commercially aware. In body-in-white there is always an element of subjective judgement.'

According to Colin Walters, the Director of Manufacturing at Peugeot-Talbot, the achieved level of flexibility at the Stoke machining plant was 'simply terrific'. He claimed, for example, that fork-lift truck drivers and inspectors also work on the machines. On the craft maintenance front, he said, mechanical fitters will also do some electrical work. He also suggests that the multi-skilling idea of creating a super-skilled, super-flexible A+ grade actually originated in manufacturing.

In sum, with regard to the issue of the flexible utilization of labour, one of our continuing themes was again borne out namely that even though most of the case companies were taking some initiatives in this direction these endeavours often did not translate into a markedly changed employment pattern. This again illustrating the point that 'strategies' and 'patterns of relations' should not be conflated.

Recruitment and Selection

Apart from developments in human resource planning and developments in forms of labour utilization there have also been changes in resourcing practices with respect to recruitment and selection. As skill shortages began to bite — especially in London and the South East - employers began to treat recruitment and retention as a priority issue. To a considerable extent the wider pattern of flexible hours, of part-time working and the like, has been a response to supply-side factors rather than simply a shift in employment strategy from the demand side. Many of the case organizations, in their Southern locations in particular, were thus experimenting with non-standard hours and recruitment of older workers and were offering special terms to encourage women to return from child-rearing.

Among measures designed to attract and retain staff these organizations have also begun consciously to design and emphasize their training and development provision. In the graduate recruitment war in particular, the relative attractiveness of rival career-development programmes has begun to figure as perhaps the most crucial weapon in the armoury. If only for this reason, certain elements of the human resource management package have increasingly come to the fore. In order to compete for labour, companies had to demonstrate some provision for training and for career-development opportunities. Additionally, they supplemented these measures with others which were equally designed to signal that they nurture their human resource in some special way or could at least give it added value on the external labour market.

Other innovative ways to retain valued staff have, according to the media, mushroomed in recent times. With competition for able people increasing and the supply of young people decreasing, employers were reported as becoming more imaginative in devising new schemes to maintain some hold over capable employees. Career break schemes (which allow women to take periods of leave of up to five years to have children) and job sharing were just two examples of the kind of initiatives which attracted attention. Innovations of this kind were accordingly looked for in the 15 case companies. A few examples were uncovered but it has to be said that they were on a very limited scale and their impact was insignificant.

Developments in the realm of selection did, however, lend some support to those who propound the human resource management thesis. A key feature here has been the increase in testing designed explicitly to assess behavioural and attitudinal characteristics. The extent, however, to which these more sophisticated and systematic approaches can be, and are, deployed depends on the sector circumstances and on the kind of wider employment-management policies being pursued. In manufacturing, for example, psychometric testing of the kind marketed by management consultants such as Saville and Holdsworth, was found to have increased significantly. The motor companies. Jaguar and Peugeot-Talbot, were both using these tests in selecting foremen and even hourly paid workers. At Jaguar, psychometric tests were designed around dimensions such as 'independence of thought', 'team working' and 'cooperativeness'. The test batteries comprise over 100 multiple-choice questions and scores out of 10 were drawn up for each. The company encountered some resistance from the unions, however, to the proposal to draw upon current employees as a means of developing the appropriate 'profile'. The idea was to profile the 'better employees' as distinct from those regarded as merely 'ordinary and below average'.

Peugeot-Talbot uses assessment centres for selecting new supervisors and for the sales and marketing workforce. Its use of Saville and Holdsworth and their Occupational Personality Questionnaire (OPQ) test has, however, been more cautious than in the case of Jaguar. While personality and attitude testing was used extensively for management and some staff grades, testing for operatives was mainly confined to reasoning ability and mechanical aptitude: Nonetheless, Peugeot-Talbot and other case companies were watching developments at Jaguar with great interest. Devices such as 'biodata', which uses an extended application form to glean a mass of detail about a candidate's 'biographical history' for matching with an 'idealized profile', were beginning to figure in the selection literature at this time. These too were tested out In the main they were not found to be making much headway. The case companies were pursuing a rather different tack - one which is designed to facilitate greater systematization and reliability in the perennially most-favoured' selection method: the interview.

The key development here was the increased use of consultant-provided packages which offer a method, and the training support, to improve the selection process without abandoning the interview - indeed these programmes retain the interview at centre stage. The packages essentially involve training over a two-to-three-day period for line managers. They promise the tools to render the process less subjective. Extensive and highly structured documentation and role-play training promise to refocus the selector's attention away from the facility with which the interviewee expresses an abstract opinion and onto actual past behaviours and supposed 'typical-behaviour' responses to a variety of stimuli.

Whichever particular technique was being used by these companies, the underlying point is that more companies seem to be following the lead publicly made so evident by Nissan (IRRR 1986: 379; Wickens 1987) and other Japanese companies (White and Trevor, 1983). While workforces are certainly much reduced there would now appear to be more care taken in the selection of that reduced employee stock. Behavioural and attitudinal characteristics are playing an increasing part in this. An inference that might be drawn from this increasing resort to systematic selection techniques is that there is some expectation that a workforce could gradually be constructed which, would be more receptive to the broad span of HR philosophy than is the case with existing manpower stocks.

The picture, overall, in the case companies concerning selection was that a number of them had launched initiatives which promised more systematic selection and a number had also set about trying to test for 'appropriate' attitudinal behavioural characteristics in their future workforces. Even among the remaining case companies, that is the ones without the psychometric tests and the like, there was evidence that they were addressing the selection issue with a new seriousness. As a corporate-level manager from the ultra-pragmatic Smith & Nephew Company put it: 'I don't know about special techniques but we have without doubt given far more attention to the selection process in recent years and here I also include the work we have done in weeding out the underperformers'.

LEADERSHIP AND MOTIVATION

Under this heading are grouped activities in the realms of:

- communication
- goal-setting, appraisal and pay
- participation and involvement.

The concept of 'leadership' or, 'managerial leadership' enjoyed a revival in the 1980s. The case companies, even those in traditional sectors, were showing a great deal of interest in it. Much of the stimulus could be traced to the influential work of Tom Peters (1985; 1987). The human resource levers associated with this were communication; goal setting, appraisal, and reward; and devices designed to elicit 'involvement'.

Communication

While communication might, on the face of it, appear to be at the 'soft' end of the continuum of initiatives it could prove to be one of the most significant. Where the expectation is built-up that each line manager will be engaged in direct communication with the workforce on a regular basis, this in itself may stimulate a need to formulate messages of substance. The activity also impels a revision of expectations about the managerial role.

What evidence is there of change in this regard? It would appear that many companies have made a step-change approach to this subject. This company prides itself on its employee communications. As the figure reveals, it has certainly installed a whole gamut of devices. The briefing meetings have now been running regularly for five years. To assist them the supervisors who are at the 'front line' of the briefing system, are provided with professionally produced briefing sheets and they have also been given training in holding team briefing sessions. 'Employee reports' and the annual financial report have been markedly upgraded and the result has been a regular series of prizes in intercompany competitions. The Ryton plant also has its own video studio and this is used to produce videos on a range of company-related topics.

The device which these companies undoubtedly saw as pivotal was the face-to-face form usually known as 'team briefing' or 'briefing groups'. This involves the first-line manager in regular and systematic meetings with his or her subordinates. In terms of the absolute number of companies which had introduced devices of this kind, the results were impressive. Direct communication to employees using line briefing was taking place in 14 out of 15 of the case companies. This finding accords with the survey of Britain's largest companies and public sector organizations undertaken in 1987 by the employee communications consultants, Vista. They found, in a survey of 222 organizations, that 86 per cent had installed a system of team briefing and 59 per cent claimed that it reached beyond the supervisory grades to all levels of staff. The Industrial Society could claim much credit for spreading the message. It had helped to introduce the system to some 400 to 500 organizations between 1984 and 1986 and many of the 15 case organizations had themselves consulted the Industrial Society for this purpose.[1]

Using the 15 company case research, it was soon revealed, however, that the real issue was not whether an organization 'had team briefing' but whether and how it was used in practice, and with what coverage across the organization. The case research suggested there were difficulties on each of these fronts. For example, it was rare to find a case where the system was being uniformally applied in practice. There were usually whole departments where briefings had not successfully taken root. The initiative in the unionized settings was also complicating collective relations. The shop stewards were in some instances rather better informed than the first line supervisors who were supposed to be giving the briefings. These supervisors said they felt exposed in transmitting a brief about topics where they might be challenged and be made to look foolish. This was particularly a complaint made by supervisors in British Rail for example. In about half a dozen of the cases the trade unions had sought to oppose the introduction of team briefings on the grounds that it was, they said, designed to bypass union channels. And of course it was. Though this was not usually its sole or main purpose.

Another development in the case companies was the practice of a certain number of key senior line managers of making direct presentations to whole departments of staff. Notable examples were at Ford Motor Company and Plessey. Works managers, plant managers and certain area managers seem to have found a confidence and competence to appeal direct to the workforce. In the instances cited, the shop stewards and conveners appeared to welcome, or at least gave grudging acknowledgement of the effectiveness of, these performances.

Goal Setting, Appraisal and Pay

Staff appraisal had typically been around in some form in most of these companies for a long time. And with equal typicality the systems had fallen into relative if not, complete disuse. What was clearly evident in the 1986-87 period, however, was the renewed interest in revising and relaunching these schemes. For managerial employees, the new fascination with appraisal was in part linked to the vogue for defining managerial 'competences'. A number of the case companies were trying to construct their own organization-specific lists. These were normally used in assessment centres for selection into management and for developmental purposes. They were also frequently found, however, being used as check-lists in appraisal and report documentation.

An approach to appraisal which was also gaining favour was built around objective setting. The key development here was the increased insistence upon *measurable* targets. In this way this aspect of managerial appraisal was increasingly being linked to another — that is, performance-related pay. During the period under review, the traditional hesitancy about linking reward to appraisal was being shrugged aside. A further feature was the extension of the appraisal device from the confines of the managerial grades to supervisors, staff and, in a few cases, to hourly paid employees. Earlier survey work (Long, 1986) had suggested that it was part of a wider trend. The proportion of companies using appraisal for manual employees had increased from a mere 2 per cent in 1977 to 24 per cent in 1986. However, the evidence from the 15 case studies would suggest a need for caution in interpreting these figures. In instances where these mainstream companies were using appraisal for hourly paid employees it was on an 'experimental' basis and its coverage in the organizations was limited to only a very small percentage of the total workforce. For example, Smith & Nephew were talking about 'trials' in the past three to four years. The

Birmingham factory had launched an elaborate scheme from a standing start. But it broke down. I don't think the MD was sufficiently clear about what he was trying to achieve' (senior S & N manager). Across the company, each division had its own particular system or non-system as the case may be. In certain divisions it was very evident that the nominal appraisal system was not taken at all seriously; a number of managers interviewed admitted they had effectively allowed it to lapse. At Plessey Naval Systems, performance appraisal for the manual grades was proposed in 1986. The scheme involved awarding discretionary 'uplifts' within the existing grade structure and these uplifts would have been consolidated into monthly salary. After three such supplements a regarding would be considered. During the research period, however, the plan was rejected by the EETPU.

Across the cases as a whole there was a definite interest in extending appraisal. It was seen as a logical tool commensurate with the moves towards harmonized terms and conditions with staff grades. Clear examples were found in parts of Whitbread. It fits also with the general aspiration to incorporate all sections of the workforce into an 'enterprise-commitment'. Individual appraisal, which could be used to set targets, monitor performance against targets, to counsel and to develop, was widely viewed as a vital tool of 'managerial leadership' which must eventually be made operable at all levels. The desire to reward individual performance also acts as a spur to further use of appraisal. Perhaps not surprisingly therefore it was also found that a key thrust in the changes to employment management so far as personnel specialists were concerned, was the drive to break at least partially away from collective pay arrangements and to introduce some variations based on individual performance.

Where individual merit payments have been installed in

the mainstream companies this was often associated with the withdrawal of bargaining recognition from managerial groups. For example, the 1988 merit-based award in BR effectively put the managers union, TSSA, outside of the bargaining process for middle management grades. And in the, NHS, the system of performance-related pay has steadily been rolled down from the most senior levels to embrace a wider and wider pool of staff. It is worth remembering that the encouragement of performance related pay and a departure from the annual pay round was part of the government's agenda of the day. Indeed, the merits of linking pay to profits as advanced by Professor Weitzman was echoed by the then Chancellor Lawson and floated in a Green Paper.

A further development in pay systems was associated with changes to long-standing pay-bargaining structures. For example, the decentralization of pay bargaining at Lucas and the announcement by BR that it was going to withdraw from the 1956 Machinery were designed to align pay with particular market circumstances. Depending on the company, these circumstances may be geographical-based, occupational-based or, ultimately, can arise from the differential competitive performance of the separated units. This last point would apply rather more to the individual businesses in a company such as Lucas Industries, but the same concept underlay the proposed shift in bargaining arrangements in British Rail. As a BR manager argued when declaring withdrawal from national bargaining : 'the many existing levels of consultation and negotiation mean that individual and local issues are often not dealt with quickly enough in the competitive climate in which the railway operates'. In other words, the intention was to allow most matters to be dealt with by local managers. In the event, of course, these proposals became a key issue in the 1989 dispute with the unions and BR was forced to trim its aspirations in this regard — at least for the time being.

Involvement

The final subsection relating to the theme of 'leadership and motivation" concerns employee involvement. Again it was soon found that a large proportion of the case organizations was taking some steps seemingly designed to encourage a measure of direct participation and involvement. Perhaps of all the devices associated with HRM that of 'quality circles' has occasioned the most comment, the most inflated expectation and the most cynicism.

The essence of the idea of quality circles is built on the twin facets of group dynamics and involvement in problem solving. The first element gives momentum: it allows diverse skills to be tapped, encourages a measure of simple fun, and it provides an audience for the demonstration of effective performance. The second element is pursued through a structured training programme in basic problem-solving techniques including, for example, brainstorming, problem identification, data collection, data analysis, cause-and-effect analysis and presentation skills. The two elements clearly potentially reinforce each other. In order to take advantage of the concept it is not necessary to abide strictly by the 'rules' of the pure QC format — though some consultants tend to argue that any *ad hoc* departures spell danger. Nonetheless, there are clearly many instances where 'problem solving groups' and 'performance-excellence teams' are operating without the QC tag. Despite the (frequently deserved) charges of faddism' attaching to QCs, the underlying concept is undoubtedly prevalent in the case companies and it remains, for them, an attractive path.[2]

Nonetheless, many of the case companies had experienced considerable difficulty in launching and sustaining quality circles. The motor companies in particular were very keen to see them succeed and yet were also faced with some of the toughest opposition: much of it deriving from TGWU national policy. Austin Rover had made a determined effort. It had used external consultants, appointed a QC coordinator and facilitator and, had trained dozens of circle leaders. But, at the time of the study, after some 18 months of manoeuvering, only 20 circles had been successfully started. Moreover, none of these was in the main target areas: the two large assembly buildings at Longbridge. Jaguar has enjoyed more acclaim for its involvement of the workforce, but even here the record was not so very different from that at Austin Rover. Indeed, the cases were remarkably alike: there had been a similar degree of managerial effort and the same kind of patchwork response. Hence, in Jaguar also, the main car-assembly buildings had remained QC free. Peugeot-Talbot had pushed less hard. A quality control programme in the early 1980s was aborted but significantly, 'problem-solving groups', which amount to much of the same thing, have been installed with some success. 'Involvement' at Peugeot-Talbot is now described as mainly the responsibility of each individual area manager. One of these had led the way by introducing visual aids such as blackboards and easels, cartoons and drawings into his area. This met with some success including, for example, the volunteering by members of this area to spend some of their own time promoting cars at the annual UK Motor Show and at various dealerships.

Ford Motor Company, while keeping a close watching brief on these other cases, have not themselves so far attempted to introduce quality circles.

At. Eaton Limited, the gearbox manufacturer, QCs had been running reasonably successfully for nearly four years. The circles were found to be meeting weekly for one hour in paid time and the company had a lengthy record of completed projects under its belt. But even here, in what must be considered one of the more, successful exemplars of QCs in operation, it was evident that continued cooperation by the workforce and the stewards was contingent upon satisfactory industrial relations on a wider front. Thus, for example, during the annual wage negotiations, the operation of circles was suspended as the adversarial character of relations became more salient. This record of union opposition stands in contrast to the experience of Plessey Naval Systems at Newport. Here, quality circles had been introduced by the factory manager but they had been 'killed off' by middle managers who saw in them a threat to their own role. The ASTMS representatives claimed that the technicians especially had welcomed the opportunity to spread their wings and they further suggested that the union representatives were broadly in favour of QCs.

If one looks beyond QCs and problem-solving teams the state of play on 'employee involvement' is, if anything, even more uncertain. The enduring impression was that managers were increasingly of the view that it was a 'good idea' but specific initiatives were hard to uncover. Joint consultative arrangements, despite their continued appearance in survey results, were rarely given much credence by line managers. The predominant desire seemed to be for some vibrant form of task-based involvement. Even the overtly cautious Smith & Nephew company decided to give a corporate-level impetus to employee involvement of this kind. The central 'IR Advisory Group', comprising the MDs of all the divisions, championed the idea and tried to impel it and to monitor its progress, but, in the absence of clear guidelines the outturn appeared insubstantial.

TRAINING AND DEVELOPMENT

It might be argued that the amount of training and development has to be the main litmus test of whether HRM has made head-way in the British context. Sisson (1989) has argued that training and development are crucial, for it is not simply that the organization which fails to train will find itself dependent upon the external labour market and thus hardly in a position to regard its workforce as anything other than a cost. The organization that does train is more likely to engage in the other, complementary, aspects of HRM — if only to protect its investment. Moreover, the training company is also more likely to be able to draw symbolic value from its actions. It is sending a message that it values its employees and they are to be viewed as an important resource and this carries the potential to structure positive attitudes across a broader front.

If this really is the crucial test of the seriousness of mainstream British organizations to the full-blown HRM model, then it has to be said that few would pass it. Survey after survey has reiterated the point that on any comparative measure, the training record of British companies has been lamentable (NEDO, 1984; Handy, 1987; Constable and McCormick, 1987). While leading employers in West Germany, Japan and the USA spend up to 3 per cent of turnover per annum on training, the comparable statistic in Britain is only around 0.15 per cent. In the lead-up to the new Training Bill in 1988, however, the government began to suggest that the situation in Britain was not so dire as these kind of figures would imply.

There were also a number of independent assessments which hinted at a more optimistic outlook, at least at the organizational level in some special cases (Keep, 1989). In a patchy way this picture was reflected in the case companies. For instance, Jaguar cars had invested heavily in the system of 'open learning'. This was designed to encourage all employees to spend some time using company facilities to engage in self-development. But as this was widely regarded as a special case the important question is what were the other companies doing with respect to training and development? Does the macro-record of lamentable under-provision find echo here or are there new signs of change?

In fact, training and development practices were found to vary tremendously in the organizations studies. In many cases the dismal underprovision catalogued by the major surveys was clearly evident. Even the sporadic training that did take place was often dismissed as inadequate. For example, a Smith and Nephew manager spoke for many when he said:

> Up to this year I've had no training whatsoever! The occasional in-company courses I've been on since then, such as presentation skills and chairmanship, have come too late.

And yet, sporadically, one encountered line managers in most of these companies who were receiving extensive training. Naturally, there was a degree of bias in the sample of managers whom one met. Those actively engaged in training and with promising career prospects tended to offer themselves forward for meetings, or, one was steered towards them because they were lively, informative and enthused. In these cases the range and impact of the training and development experiences often proved to be impressive.

Among the main case companies the revamped training practices at Lucas Industries probably represented one of the more dramatic and convincing instances of across the board upgrading of training provision. In fact, Lucas has had an above average training record for many decades, but what is interesting about this case is the way in which the training had been revitalized during a very difficult period of restructuring and divestment in the 1980s.

Senior management contend that organizational transformation at Lucas had been driven by a rigorous 'systems engineering' approach. This, it will be recalled, has three elements;

- new technology
- alterations to the organizational system (most notably a devolution to strategic business units)
- new methods including, for example, Kanban and Just-In-Time.

The buttress to each of these three, is 'a really major effort in training'. Indeed, at one meeting with corporate chiefs it was claimed that 'we are doing 50 times what Jaguar are doing'. The strategic place of training and development at Lucas stems from the intent to move radically from the standardization and divisionalization of the 1960s and 1970s 'which may have been appropriate at that time but certainly not so now', according to Dr John Parnaby, Group Director Manufacturing Technology. The new competitive conditions are seen as putting a premium on versatility. Under such circumstances 'our aim' said Parnaby, 'is not to substitute a new "method" but rather to help our managers and staff learn principles so that they can be innovative in their own setting. Local teams have to create their own solutions.' These teams in each of the 135 separate businesses can, if they wish, call on the assistance of a corporate 'task force'. At the end of the day, however, the SBUs are held responsible: Lucas operates on a 'loose-tight' principle using a combination of persuasion and pressure. Training has played a vital part in driving this strategy.

In the period 1985-8, Lucas has spent around £40m per annum on training which was equivalent to about 2.5—3 per cent of its total sales revenue. This expenditure was viewed as an 'investment' in that training and development was being called on to act as a major agent of change. The in-company consciousness of the key role of training was high. It was not seen as a poor-relation, peripheral activity, but as a potent source of change. The highlights of the contribution made by training in this company are:

- its link with the total strategy comprising marketing, product engineering, manufacturing systems engineering and business systems
- the highly evident top management commitment to it
- its role in developing and executing the competitive achievement plans (CAPs) which every business unit is required to have
- the installation of business and engineering systems into the SBUs
- and the underpinning of business task forces through training on an essentially project-requirement basis.

At the core of the Lucas turnaround strategy is the the transformation of Lucas manufacturing systems. As Parnaby observed:

> competitiveness to world standards requires a fundamental redesign of our manufacturing systems and farreaching changes in traditional working practices, habits and culture. Our most potent engines of change are the multidisciplinary task forces which operate mainly at business unit and factory level. Once the members of each task force have been given basic training in systems engineering, they then redesign their factory or business units on the basis of 'Just-In-Time' control systems.... they develop plans for marketing their products, improving quality, changing job structures, improving the performance of their suppliers and not feast training all the people in the business unit.

This programme is so extensive that he estimated that by 1991 just about the whole of the workforce would undergo some form of training. (The fact that this was considered extraordinary even in a major training company such as this indicates the distance British organizations have to cover.) The delivery mechanisms included, in addition to the task force methodology, an active central training function which has reoriented itself from training delivery to training development; open learning centres; modular courses in manufacturing systems; and external masters courses.

The Lucas case provides an excellent example of a traditional, mainstream company which, in seeking to turn itself around from a loss-making situation, has sought a radical strategic response part of which has clearly involved a drive to enhance the capabilities and commitment of its human resources through the use of training.

And yet the Lucas case is at the same time, instructive for another reason. Its training provision especially its coherent, business-led analysis of the role of that provision is distinctive for its singularity. Few companies and this includes the rest of the cases involved in this project could claim to match the emphasis upon human resource development which has been shown by Lucas. But despite this lead position, it has to be said that only a little digging around is required to reveal that the impact, when viewed from the stance of the intended recipients of such provision, is, even in this lead case, often minimal. The approach looks coherent, sophisticated and integrated when presented by senior exponents, but it is often experienced rather differently by shopfloor workers and indeed by many middle-level managers. Both groups relate how their own recent training experiences have been few and how the investment-in-people theme is countermanded by more visible messages of cost cutting and pressure.

To note these negative responses is by no means to mark out Lucas for any particular criticism. The point extends well beyond such an exercise. What the case illustrates, is indeed, the extreme difficulty of formulating and implementing an HRM approach in part or in whole in the context of traditional businesses in Britain which not only inherit whole congeries of expectations and past practices but which, at the same time, have also been facing harsh competitive pressures. In this light, it may be seen that the difficulties encountered at Lucas though their achievements should of course not as a consequence, be neglected are reflective of a much wider set of problems which seem to be impeding the progress of human resource management in the UK.

SUMMARY

The chapter opened with a summary overview of the results from the 15 case studies. This revealed that, at least in broad terms, there *did* appear to be evidence of extensive managerial initiatives across the critical dimensions which had been identified in earlier chapters. It was recognized, however, that these results were only a pictorial representation of apparent change and that to be meaningful they required deeper exploration. This chapter commenced that task by examining developments in three main areas: resourcing and utilization; leadership and motivation; and training and development. The overall trend was incontrovertibly towards more individualized arrangements. Many of the particular devices had a rather patchy application but the pressure was found to be continuing in this direction. The basic tenets of HRM would seem to be enjoying some wide appeal among managers if only in furnishing an aspiration and a sense of direction. The crucial importance of symbolism in helping to conjure the nature of that goal was very evident.

While examining different realms of initiative this chapter reveals that there is by no means a uniform pattern of practice. Significant changes in such spheres as selection, training, flexible working and communication had clearly been driven some distance by case companies such as Jaguar, Lucas and Ford. But other cases such as Plessey and Smith & Nephew suggested a limited degree of change. And yet, what is also of some import is that in practically all of the 15 cases, the senior line managers were of a broadly common mind regarding the direction in which they wanted to travel and the kinds of changes they would like to see. The symbolic function of HRM in this regard was that it helped to provide some measure of logic to a host of often disparate initiatives. Hence, arguably, it was not the nature or content of employment management practices that was in particular contention but rather the process and feasibility of how to achieve the desired ends. It is to this issue of change processes that we now turn.

NOTES

1 Where there is some legislative requirement, however, one might expect rather firmer monitoring. Section 1 of the 1982 Employment Act obliges companies with more than 250 employees to include in their annual reports a statement describing action taken to inform, consult and involve their employees. This provision came into effect in 1985. In June of that year the Employment Minister reported on a survey conducted by the Department of Employment on compliance with this section. The survey revealed 15 per cent did not report in accordance with the requirement. A further 40 per cent acknowledged the legal requirement but gave little or no detail of what they were doing. Of the remaining 45 per cent which did report, the largest proportion listed share schemes as their method of 'involvement', closely followed by company newspapers and line briefings (31 per cent of those surveyed). A broadly similar set of findings emerged from the ACAS/LBS (1986) survey of 300 company reports. This study emphasizes however, that the findings relate to what company report claim is being done, and these claims do not necessarily accord with what is actually happening.

2 Because of the difficulties of definition it is almost impossible to quantify the extent of operation of such groups. The National Society of Quality Circles (NSQC) which was launched in Britain

in 1982 had 260 companies in full membership in early 1989: these included star names such as ICI, Barclays, Nat West, Tioxide and Rowntrees. It is estimated that there are some 5000 to 6000 circles functioning across the UK. The NSQC shrugs off scepticism about 'flavour of the month' by pointing to the "marked increase in inquiries' throughout 1988 and early 1989. In January 1989 they were said to be running at 12 -15 company enquiries per week (personal communication).

10

HUMAN RESOURCE MANAGEMENT

"They who boast most, generally fail most, for deeds are silent."
—*An Old Proverb*

It has been established by recent studies that the Human Resource Management policies are influenced by two major considerations: Situational factors and Stakeholder interests. Situational factors are those forces—laws and societal values, labour market conditions, unions, work-force characteristics, business strategies, management philosophy, and task technology—that exist in the environment or inside the firm. Situational factors can act as constraints on the HRM policies formation and can also be influenced by HRM policies. HRM policies are and indeed should be influenced by the interests of various stakeholders: shareholders, unions, management employees, community, and government. If these policies are not influenced by all stakeholders, the enterprise will fail to meet the needs of these stakeholders in the long run.

Policy choices made by managers affect the overall competence of employees, the commitment of employees, the degree of congruence between the goals of employees and those of the organization, and the overall cost effectiveness of HRM practices. These four Cs are not exhaustive of the criteria that HRM policy makers may find useful in evaluating the effectiveness of human resource management, but they are reasonably comprehensive.

HRM policy choices affect the four Cs and have long-term consequences for individual well-being, organizational effectiveness, and societal well-being. But long-term consequences also affect situational factors and stakeholder interests. For examble, strikes that affect society negatively can influence changes in labour legislation. Poor profitability over an extended period will affect shareholder interest and must inevitably result in changes of HRM policies regarding wages, training. There are other feedback effects also. The central point is that the long-term consequences of HRM policies for individual well-being, organizational effectiveness, and societal well-being will affect those policies and the context within which these are formulated.

As a central matter, to clarify who has a stake in the issue at hand, to identify these stakes, and to determine how much power they may be able to apply. These questions are analytically important whether the decision-maker ultimately wants to accommodate or deny the interests of another stakeholder. One can use other aspects of the analytical framework in various ways. If managers want to understand why their company is currently pursuing a particular approach to an HRM issue, such as an adversarial stance toward labour relations they must analyze the situational factors, both their current force and their influence in the past.

Managers may want to compare the relevant merits of two HRM policy alternatives, such as a work system with narrowly defined jobs versus one emphasizing whole tasks and team responsibilities. These managers can then attempt to forecast the differential effects of the two systems on the development of competence, the level of commitment, and the like. They can also attempt to extend the forecast another step by asking how good each policy is for the enterprise, the individual, and society.

Managers must also examine the question of fit among HRM policies—specifically the fit of the policy being reviewed with the other HRM policies and systems.

Evaluation of HRM Policies

We have proposed that the long-term consequences of HRM policies be evaluated in terms of their benefits and costs at three levels: the individual, the organization, and society.

Basically, it is almost tautological to argue that an organization's HRM policies should be evaluated in terms of whether they promote the organization's goal achievement and survival. An HRM policy may be important because it serves to increase the organization's efficiency or its adaptability, its service performance or its price performance, its short-term results or its long-term results. The well-being of employees must be a separate and distinct consideration. Working conditions can have both positive and negative effects not only on employees' economic welfare, but on their physical and psychological health. The amount of weight managers will choose to give to such consequences.

Notably, evaluation of HRM results can also be made on the *societal level.* Alienated and laid-off workers may develop both psychological and physical health problems that make them burdens to community agencies funded by the local, state, or federal government. Today employers pass on many of the costs of their management practices to society. Whoever bears these costs, they should be recognized as associated with the HRM policy decisions made by management. In some areas there is a near coincidence of interests between corporations, individuals, and society.

In considering whether an HRM policy enhances the performance of the organization, the well-being of employees, or the well-being of society, the four Cs can be taken in to account.

1. *Commitment.* Increased commitment can result not only in more loyalty and better performance for the organization, but also in self-worth, dignity, psychological involvement, and identity for the individual.
2. *Competence.* When needed skills and knowledge are available at the right time, the organization benefits and its employees experience an increased sense of self-worth and economic well-being. Data about employee commitment can be obtained by managers in any area of the organization by means of attitude surveys. These surveys can be conducted through interviews and questionnaires administered either by personnel specialists or by outside consultants. Open-door policies and observations of group meetings with employees can also keep managers in touch with their employees' attitudes.
3. *Cost effectiveness.* Such costs can be considered for organizations, individuals, and society as a whole policy. Cost effectiveness may appear to be easier to measure, but that appearance can be deceiving. Wages are the easiest to assess, while the long-term costs of certain profit-sharing plans, pension plans, and cost-of-living adjustments are more difficult to assess because of future uncertainties. The cost effectiveness of recruitment and employee development is even more difficult to measure, yet both are an important part of the total employment cost.
4. *Congruence.* The lack of congruence can be costly to management in terms of time, money, and energy, in terms of the resulting low levels of trust and common

purpose, and in terms of stress and other psychological problems it can create. Congruence of goals can be more easily identified, particularly when its absence results in an open conflict like a strike. Although the total costs of a strike are difficult to pin down, such an assessment can be part of a total assessment of HRM policies.

It should be remembered that, the four 'Cs' do not provide managers with actual measurement methods and data for assessing the effects of their firm's HRM policies. These methods are numerous, and they differ depending on the level of analysis chosen (individual, corporation, or society). Corporations gather data on the competence of employees through performance evaluation by managers and through third-party assessment of competence by personnel specialists, psychologists, other managers, or assessment centers.

Another source of data—personnel records about voluntary turnover, absenteeism, and grievances—can provide indirect evidence about employee commitment. Taken together, such data might fall short of providing managers with an absolute measure of commitment and congruence, but they can provide a useful overall picture.

These difficulties in measurement are exceeded by the difficulties in making judgments about consequences of HRM policies on employee and societal well-being. Various governance mechanisms such as union-management task forces or employee committees can provide important vehicles not only for gathering data about human resource outcomes, but for assessing the meaning of these outcomes for various stakeholders. Workers council and collective bargaining are examples of legislated governance mechanisms that serve the same purpose.

The desire to account for human resources as if they

were in the same metric as financial resources has led to experimentation with human resource accounting systems. These systems have tried to value a person by estimating his or her replacement costs and the investment the firm has made in that person's recruitment, training, and development. Such accounting efforts, while potentially very useful, have fallen short of their promise, at least judging by the fact that they are not widely used. An even more difficult task has been assigning a value to the commitment of employees or the climate and culture of the firm which encourage motivation and growth by its employees. These difficulties are not likely to be overcome soon. In the final analysis, assessment of HRM outcomes is a matter of judgment informed by data from a variety of sources and in a variety of forms (qualitative and quantitative) and evaluated by various stakeholders.

Stakeholder Interest

Stakeholders in a given enterprise may include owners, government, host communities, workers, labour unions, and the manager themselves. Different employee groups can have different stake in a particular policy matter. Younger and older workers might find their interests affected in very different ways by company policies relating to benefits and pensions. So might male and female employees. In general employees and management will surely differ with some frequency over such matters as the amount and kind of pay, benefits, and conditions of work. While these are rewards to employees, they are costs to the employer—costs that reduce profits and investment funds.

Why are workers not as concerned as management about corporate profits? Why shouldn't they be more self-regulating in their expectations and demands for monetary and nonmonetary rewards? And why are managers not more understanding about worker needs and more concerned about worker well-being in their decisions? The answers lie, in part, in the different interests of the two groups. Those groups often have different views about the necessary but sometimes difficult trade-offs made within an organization—trade-offs between business goals of efficiency, growth, and investment on the one hand and employee needs for security, equity, job satisfaction, and economic well-being on the other.

The task of general managers is to recognize the potential for differing—even conflicting—points of view among the various stakeholders over how trade-offs should be made. They must develop a role and perspective that allows them to manage the trade-off process in such a way as to minimize differences between stakeholders and to contain conflict when it arises. For American managers such a role represents quite a departure from the traditionally espoused shareholder perspective. While in actuality managers already manage in a way that recognizes shareholders as only one among many groups of stakeholders, conscious acceptance of the stakeholder perspective would put them in an even more neutral position with respect to shareholders to whom they traditionally have felt accountable. Given the make-up of boards of directors and the power of financial institutions, adopting a stakeholder perspective as opposed to shareholder perspective could be very difficult.

Situational Factors

The HRM model suggests that HRM policies and practices must be designed and implemented to fit a variety of important situational factors. HRM policies should be *contingent* on situational factors, or that they become the dependent variable. To the contrary, in the long run, all situational factors are subject to some influence by creative HRM policies and practices. Some situational factors are subject to influence by HRM policies in the short to medium term. The use of the term "situational factors" should not imply that these factors are all "outside" the firm. Clearly, unions, laws, societal values, and labor markets are external to the firm in the sense that they are part of the organization's environment; yet they emerge, in part at least, from the human resource policies of the past. Management philosophy, work-force characteristics, task technology, and business strategy are "inside" the firm in the sense that they appear to be subject to more managerial control, yet they are also affected by external business and societal forces.

Work-Force Characteristics

Managers at every level and in every function of the organization convey their answer to this question through their managerial actions: corporations convey their answer through their HRM policies and practices. These policies and practices reflect the *assumptions* of management about employee motivation, capacities, values, potential, and desire for personal development. If the assumptions are not consistent with reality or potential of the work force, HRM policies and practices will not fully utilize or develop employees, resulting in potential loss for both employers and employees. In addition, such policies may create conflict between employees and the organization.

To simplify the problem of fitting policies to work-force characteristics, corporations typically develop different HRM policies and practices for different groups of employees. Administratively, the work force in most U.S. corporations is typically broken down into four identifiable aggregates: (1) hourly and blue-collar, (2) nonexempt salaried white-collar, (3) exempt salaried professionals, and (4) managers. Within these groupings, of course, there are many meaningful sub-groupings such as engineers, clerical personnel, skilled tradespeople, younger and older workers, and so on.

Policy differences should be shaped by valid assumptions about the differences in background, needs, expectations, and educational qualifications that employees bring to their jobs. However, managers must be careful not to differentiate between groups on the basis of invalid assumptions. Distortions are most likely to occur with respect to people at lower levels of the organization. In part at least, policy differences between groups have arisen because managers make assumptions that lower-level people—who are different from them in terms of background, social skills, and values—lack the will and skill to contribute and the potential to develop. This distortion can happen easily because today's managers are often isolated from nonmanagerial employees by organizational practices, hierarchy, and bureaucracy. Managers are no longer promoted from hourly ranks as they once were. Rather, they are educated in business schools where their main contacts are with other prospective managers.

The problem of emphasizing differences rather than similarities is most acute with respect to ethnic minorities and women in the work force.

Business Strategy and Conditions

An organization's HRM policies and practices must fit with its strategy in its competitive environment and with the immediate business conditions that it faces. If a manufacturing firm operates in a highly competitive environment in which cost effectiveness and efficiency in manufacturing are key, that firm needs to develop HRM policies and practices that encourage cost savings efforts by all its employees. If quality is a key success factor, then HRM policies and practices must encourage concern and involvement of employees with the quality problem. If a professional service firm depends on attracting, motivating, and keeping the best professionals in their field, then that firm must develop HRM policies that bring in the best people, develop their competencies, and offer rewards and other inducements that encourage the right people to join and stay with the firm.

The match between HRM policies and business strategy is often poor. One reason for this is that managers often develop business plans and make capital investments without adequate regard to the human resources needed to support those plans. For example, growth plans involving the building of plants or opening of branch offices may take inadequate account of a shortage of managers to run these facilities. The result can be lower returns on investment or even complete business failures. Managers, at least those outside the HR functional area, have typically assumed that human resources are not a constraint and will be available in sufficient quality and quality. With increasing managerial and technical complexity and a scarcity of talent, that assumption is often erroneous.

That function often develops activities and programs that are not relevant to line management's needs. This problem arises in part from the differences is perspective between short-term, profit-oriented line managers and long-term, people-oriented human resource managers. But the problem also stems from the fact that many HR activities are not developed in close coordination with business planning. HR executives are often left out of the business planning process, frequently because they do not occupy a high level in the organization. Just as regularly, these executives develop policies and practices based on general assumptions about the kinds of behavior and performance required rather than on a careful analysis of the strategy, the tasks that the strategy presents to the organization, and the competencies and involvement required from employees. Business strategies can also shape the human resources of the firm, the types of people, attitudes, and commitment the firm is likely to obtain.

If a company's success rests on promoting a relatively undifferentiated consumer product through advertising and promotion, for example, it needs to attract people whose skills are quite different from those of people in a firm where technology-driven products are clearly differentiated. The latter firm is likely to have longer-range goals, and needs to attract and keep people interested in contributing to these goals. The former is likely to set much shorter-term goals and rely on people attracted to quick results and personal gains. The competencies and commitments of the two employee groups are likely to be quite different. This does not suggest that one business is more desirable than another. It does point out that product/market strategies might constrain the kind of HRM policies and outcomes possible. Since these HRM policies must also fit with management's values, those values must be understood when managers make business strategy decisions. Ideally, then, business strategy should influence HRM policies and practices.

Management Philosophy

The HRM policies of an organization are shaped by the management philosophy of its key managers, just as the philosophy of these leaders is shaped by the historical pattern of HRM policies. The relationship between HRM policies and management philosophy is stronger in some organizations than in others, depending on the pattern of development of the organization. If, in the early stages of development, an organization has a powerful founder and leader with a clearly articulated philosophy and set of values, HRM policies are more likely to be internally consistent. This consistency will create a stronger and more pervasive culture with respect to HRM matters.

"Management philosophy" is the explicit or implicit *beliefs* of key managers about the nature of the business, its role in society, and how it should be run—particularly how it will treat and utilize employees. A manager's philosophy is shaped by his or her values or assumptions about the role of business in society and the role of people in the business.

These questions, while challenging the imagination of managers in diffusing and sustaining a philosophy, in no way weaken the known link between management philosophy and HRM policies. In fact, the importance of that link has been acknowledged in recent efforts to create innovative work systems at the plant level aimed at developing high commitment among employees. These efforts typically involve the definition, in advance of plant start-up, of a philosophy of management, that will guide the design of human resource policies and practices. This process not only helps lead to a consensus among the management team about what the philosophy should be, thereby socializing them into a common view, but it also provides a guideline for future action as new events and realities unfold. Without a stated belief system, short-term pragmatic consideration would dominate HRM policy decisions rather than simply influence them. The result would be inconsistent new policies and an erosion of the philosophy. Thus, a general philosophy allows lower-level managers and future managers to shape new HRM policies and practices that are consistent with the philosophy but pragmatic and relevant to the immediate situation.

Management's philosophy, whether stated or unstated, is not the only way managers shape HRM policies and practices. Their *style* of management—the way they behave, communicate, and interact with others—sends a powerful signal up and down the organization about what they care about. It also helps to shape the organization's HRM manager policies and practices. If managers state their philosophy that employees should be given the opportunity to grow. and develop through participation in management, and then make unilateral decisions revising decisions made at a lower level, the credibility of policies that encourage worker participation may be undermined. Similarly, policies that encourage employee development through open and candid discussions of performance with subordinates are not likely to be implemented if upper level managers do not model this process through their own practices. The lack of consistency between philosophy and policies can also undermine sustained implementation of HRM policies. Managers who have formulated a policy that conflicts with their own philosophy are not likely to sustain follow-up efforts to implement that policy.

Labour Market Conditions

With respect to human resources, managerial ability is determined by the attractiveness of the company to prospective recruits and current employees, as well as the condition of the labor markets from which the firm draws its supply of people. The boundaries that define the labor markets in which a firm competes may vary dramatically from one group of employees to another. For unskilled production employees, the labor market may be the surrounding community. For professionals and managers, the labor market may encompass all professionals in that category in the nation. New hires will be motivated to come to work for a company and current employees will stay if they perceive the company's wages, location, organizational climate, advancement opportunities, job security, and working conditions as more attractive than those of other companies.

Over a period of time, these factors combine to form a firm's reputation in the several labor markets in which it competes. That reputation becomes an asset or a liability in attracting and keeping employees. For example, a firm that has a reputation for periodic force reductions may have difficulty competing for employees, particularly for employees in scarce supply.

But the ability of managers to attract and retain the people they need also depends on the conditions of labor markets in which they compete, as well as on their firm's HRM policies.

Shortages of people with given skills make it more difficult for a corporation to attract and keep people. In cases where it is extremely difficult to find people with the right skills, business plans and goals are affected. In tight labor markets, firms have to offer more inducements than they would otherwise in order to attract and keep people. Of course, the more a company is able to develop and keep its own professionals, managers, and other skilled employees, the less hiring of experienced personnel it has to do. The desire to reduce, as much as possible, the necessity of competing in a tight labor market has led some firms to consider an employment security policy. It has also led firms to intensify their efforts in training and developing their own employees.

Managers are well advised to track long-term trends in labor markets, since these trends indicate how difficult and/ or expensive it will be to acquire people with the skills their business may require in the future. Information of this kind can help managers assess the viability of their long-term strategic plans. Perhaps more important, it can point to changes that will be needed in educational programming at colleges, trade schools, and professional schools [which will be needed] to assure employers themselves of an adequate supply of people with the right skills. When shortages are indicated, firms can attempt to influence educational institutions to modify their programs and recruit more students in an effort to influence the labor market. Or, business organizations can set up their own internal educational programs. Firms in high-technology fields have been doing both as they have come to realize that there will be a shortage of electrical engineers in the 1980s. Those that recognized the trends sooner and anticipated their needs more adequately will be able to compete more effectively in the labor market and the business.

Trends in the labor market include changes in the participation of women and minorities as well as changing values of the work force that make employees more resistant to arbitrary authority. And the movement of the post-World War II "baby boom" has created a gradual aging of the work force that will place changing demands on HRM policies, particularly in the areas of flow and rewards. These trends, if not anticipated, can present real problems to managers who have not adjusted their HRM policies and practices to fit them. On the other hand, organizations that effect changes in HRM policies and practices in anticipation of demographic trends can gain a competitive advantage by being better able to attract, utilize, and keep a new breed of employee.

Unions

Historically, unions have served as a mechanism to provide a collective voice for nonsupervisory workers over such HRM matters as due process, the distribution of rewards, transfers and promotions, and working conditions. Even where employees are not unionized, unions can influence HRM policies. The perceived threat of unionization can lead employers to adopt HRM policies and practices that they might otherwise avoid. Within a company, wage increases negotiated by the union create pressures to increase wages for nonunion employees by a similar or slightly greater amount in order to avoid dissatisfaction that might lead to further union organizing. Firms without any union may feel forced to pay close attention to pay, fringe benefits, employment security, working conditions, promotion practices, and termination practices. If a corporation operates in a heavily unionized community, it must establish some degree of parity between its policies and those of unionized firms, or risk unionization.

Unions influence HRM practices of nonunionized firms indirectly through their political influence. Legislation that has come about, in large part, because of the political clout of unions has imposed certain human resource standards on employers. Occupational health and safety, workman's compensation, and minimum wage legislation are just three examples. In France and Britain, where unions are more closely allied with political parties than in the United States, their influence is even greater and is felt not only in legislation but in government policy with regard to human resource practices. Even though only 35 per cent of the U.S. work force was unionized at the peak of union power in the 1960s, unions have had an important effect on human resource policies and practices of all American businesses, unionized or not.

Task Technology

"Task technology" is the way equipment (hardware or software) is arranged to perform a task. Historically, the technology used to produce a product or provide a service has had a powerful and pervasive effect on human resource policies and practices, particularly in manufacturing operations. It has been shaped by the engineer's view of what constitutes a rational and efficient operation. That rational view has traditionally dominated plant layout and the design of jobs. Similarly, the imperatives of technology itself often have determined the nature of work. The machine and the task have tended to constitute the independent variables, while human beings were left to be the dependent variable.

This view of technology has largely shaped the nature of work as we find it in the late twentieth century. It spawned the assembly line, as well as the division of work in which "planning" and "controlling" have been systematically split off from "doing" and assigned to higher levels or staff groups. Even "doing"' has been divided still further with the goal of reducing the time and cost of employee selection and training. This trend has led to problems of depersonalization, boredom, and alienation. Such human problems may in part be responsible for the rise of unionization.

Technology is now also transforming the office. The work of clerical employees, professionals, and managers will be affected as new information technology (minicomputers and word processing, for example) is introduced and becomes an integral part of the work system for these employees.

Laws and Societal Values

HRM policies and practices in various countries differ in accordance with the unique culture or ideology of each society. By culture, we mean the values or basic assumptions that people in a society or an organization seem to hold about how one ought to think and behave. These assumptions are often implicit and can be inferred from the standards of expected behavior that are informally enforced by the society, organization, or group. These standards of expected behavior are sometimes called "norms." Ideology is a dynamic framework of interrelated values and beliefs that emerges within a society and is used by that society to make its values explicit and give them institutional validity. Thus, ideology is more explicit than culture or norms and can be found in formal statements of beliefs provided by leaders and other prominent societal and organizational members. Ideologies are modified in response to changes in the nature of a society and in the real world in which that society exists. For example, ideology is shaped by the unique historical and political development of the society, and that development is a function of realities such as geography, demography, resource availability, evolution of traditional institutions, and patterns of behavior and the collective experience of the society as it struggles to survive and prosper. The process of ideology formulation is, therefore, a dynamic one: Changes occur as the society is confronted with new realities. The importance of ideology is that it serves as a bridge between universally held values such as survival, justice, security, self-fulfillment, economic use of resources, and self-respect and the means by which those values are put into practice in a particular setting and at a particular time.

It should not be surprising that HRM policies differ across societies because of explicit differences in government policies and legislation governing employer-employee relations. With the exception of Japan, where emphasis on informal understandings and relationships reduces reliance on legislation, most countries have developed extensive legal frameworks specifying the HRM policies and practices that firms are to employ. Legislation governing employer-employee relations develops out of negative experience of employees with HRM practices in the society. These result in political pressures on government to legislate or regulate HRM practices.

Legislation affecting HRM policies and practices includes the legal framework in which unionization and union-management relations occur, wage and hour laws which govern payment of overtime, laws governing occupational health and safety, equal employment opportunity legislation, legislation governing employee pension funds, and income maintenance programs like workers compensation. In Europe, more extensive legislation exists to govern employee relations, including strict rules that restrict the freedom of management to terminate employees and legislation which establishes the rights and framework for employee participation in an enterprise. As with other legislation, of course, the intent of this legislation is quite often not translated into practice. Managers who do not accept the right of employees to participate find ways to circumvent that legislated process, just as employee representatives who do not have experience in business have some difficulty participating meaningfully, even if they have been encouraged to do so. Thus, a society that seeks to influence HRM must, over time, transform the ideology and skills of both managers and employees if real transformations are to occur.

Obviously HRM policies and practices are not and cannot be formed in a vacuum. They must reflect the governmental and societal context in which they are embedded. For this reason, policies and practices that work in the United States will not necessarily work in Europe or Japan. Similarly, Japanese multinational firms have discovered that not all policies that have been effective in their home country are applicable in the United States. Company housing, slow promotion, or promotion based on seniority, for instance, may not have the same effect outside of the Japanese context. Managers both in and out of an organization's human resource function must understand the culture, ideology, legislation, and regulations of the society in which they operate before formulating HRM policies.

Just as important, variations in HRM policies and practices across countries offer useful alternatives for U.S. managers to learn from. This comparative perspective allows managers to examine and question the ideology and assumptions that underlie their own HRM practices. Looking at what managers in other countries do can also suggest alternative models for integrating people and organizations. The interest of American managers in Japanese practices and the stimulus for change provided by the success of Japanese management are the best examples of this phenomenon. However, wholesale application of HRM policies from another country must be avoided if good fit with situational factors is to be obtained. By studying other cultures, U.S. managers may also be able to discern long-term patterns that may engulf them in the future.

Organizational Adaptability

Implicit in much of the discussion here is the assumption that effective human resource management policies and practices lead to increased adaptability, a critical ingredient in the long-term survival of business organizations. This point is discussed more explicitly below.

Organizational effectiveness in the long run means that the firm has been flexible and responsive to its market and social environment. When the market demands lower costs, or product innovation, or improved service, the management of the corporation must sense the need for change and be able to mobilize the support of various stake-holders, employee groups, unions, government, educational institutions, suppliers, and the community to make adjustments in their own expectations and behavior. Effective HRM policies and practices are those that are designed and administered through a process of mutual influence between management and employees and that result in high levels of commitment, competence, cost effectiveness, and congruence.

Here is how the four Cs can contribute to employee and organizational adaptability.

1. *High commitment* means that employees will be motivated to hear, understand, and respond to management's communications about changes in environmental demands with their implications for wages, work practices, and competency requirements. The mutual trust will be there to enable management's message to be more believable to employees and to enable management to be responsive to employee's legitimate concerns as stakeholders.
2. *High competence* means that employees in the firm will have the versatility in skills and the perspective to take on new roles and jobs as needed. Through a positive attitude toward learning and personal development fostered by policies that encourage and reward learning, employees will be more capable of responding to change.
3. *Cost effectiveness* means that the organization's human resource costs—wages, benefits, and indirect costs such as strikes, turnover, and grievances—have been kept

equal to or less than those of competitors, while major adjustments such as the ones facing employees in the steel and auto industries have been avoided. Once again, only a continual process of mutual influence about the realities of the business and the needs of employees can bring about this outcome.

4. *Higher congruence* than competitors means that the firm has shaped work systems, reward systems, and flow policies so that there is a higher coincidence of interest among management, shareholders, and workers. Furthermore, a process of employee influence in the affairs of the company will also foster congruence. In such a climate, changes in policies and practices prompted by the external environment are less likely to be perceived by employees as not in their interest. Moreover, the inevitable differences between shareholder interests and employee interests that remain in even the most effective corporations will probably be easier to manage because an atmosphere of collaboration and mutual problem solving will have been developed between stakeholders.

Managers in adaptive organizations can sense changes in societal values and attend to the spirit as well as the letter of laws that operationalize these values. These changes begin to be reflected in their management philosophy and practices, particularly their human resource practices. Managers who see themselves as responsible for the well-being of the enterprise, its employees, and society—i.e., for long-term consequences as opposed to the more narrow' outcomes such as profit or growth—are more likely to sense and incorporate changes in societal values into human resource policies. Their HRM policies are less likely to undermine their relationships with their employees, government, and community.

Summing Up

Similarly management philosophy, business strategy, labor markets, laws and society, task technology, and unions affect HR policies and to varying degrees are affected by them For many of these factors—business strategy, task technology, unions, and management philosophy—a two-way process of influence is possible and needs to be strengthened. That is, policies need to be forged with a clearer understanding of the constraints, just as those constraints may be seen as amenable to modification by progressive and well-articulated HRM policies. Other factors, such as laws, society, and labor markets, may be more immutable constraints in the short run, but even they are subject to influence and change in the long run. We characterized each of the situational factors interacting with human resource policies in the belief that a better understanding of their influence will allow managers to design policies that fit the situation and/or change the situation.

Remarkably, the interests of various stakeholders—shareholders, management, employees, government, the community, and unions—must also be an important factor in designing HRM policies and practices. Without attention to the perspectives of all stakeholders, HRM policies and priorities are unlikely to gain their acceptance. In the long run this is likely to result in the failure of those policies and in a loss of organizational effectiveness.

The well-being of the enterprise, society, and employees were suggested as long-term criteria by which general managers ought to evaluate the HRM policies of their organization. The clear implication is that general managers should search for policies that enhance the well-being of all three, not the enterprise alone, which has traditionally been the central consideration. Finally, commitment, competence, congruity, and cost effectiveness were suggested as specific outcomes that help define all three long-term criteria and that should be assessed explicitly in evaluating human resource policies. Innovative companies are explicitly shaping policies to enhance commitment, competence, and congruence, outcomes that in many companies are by-products of human resource policies rather than explicit goals. Such policy shaping increases an organization's capacity to adapt to changes in its environment.

SELECT BIBLIOGRAPHY

Ahuja, Shobha (2002) Creating Corporate Advantage through Human Resource Development. *Vision: The Journal of Business Perspective.* Jan.-June 2002, pp. 73-86.

Appelbaum, S.H. and Goransson, L. (1997) 'Transformational and adaptive learning within the learning organization: a framework for research and application', *The Learning Organization,* 4(3):115 –128.

Argyris, C. (1993) *Knowledge for Action: A Guide to Overcoming Barriers to Organizational Change,* Jossey Bass, San Francisco, CA.

Argyris, C. and Schon, D.A. (1978) *'Organisation Learning: A Theory of Action Perspective',* Reading M.A.: Addison-Wesley.

Arnopoulos, P. (1991) 'Ideological analytics: a study of evolving world values', *World Futures,* 30, 1, 19-34.

Ashley, D. (1984) 'Historical materialism and ideological practice: how do ideologies dominate people?', *Current Perspectives in Social Theory,* 5 (2): 1-20.

Ashok, J. (2003) 'Cognition, culture and competition: an empirical test of the learning organization', *The Learning Organization,*10(1): 31-50.

Barney, J.(1991) Firm Resources and Sustained Competitive Advantage. *Journal of Management,* 17: 99-129.

Bhamidipati, Ravi and Makhijani, Rajen (2003) 'Changing Mindsets', Background Papers, AIMA 30th National Management Convention, September 15-17.

Bhandarker, Asha and Singh, Pritam (2003) 'Leading to Win', Background Papers, AIMA 30th National Management Convention, September 15-17.

Bhaskar, A.U., Ratnam, C.S.V. and Bhal, K.T. (2003) Employment Relations in a Global Economy: A Paradigm Shift.

Bhat, Mushtaq A. (2003) *Service Quality in Service Sector Banks: An Empirical Investigation*, Business Review, Vol.9, No. 2, March.

Bierema, L. L. (1999). A model of executive women's learning and development. *Adult Education Quarterly*, *49*(2), 107-121.

Bing, John W., Kehrhahn, Marijka and Short, Darren C. (2003) 'Challenge to the Field of Human Resource Development', *Advances in Developing Human Resources*, Vol. 5, No. 3 August.

Birley, S. (1989). Female entrepreneurs: Are they really different? *Journal of Small Business Management*, 27(2), 32-37.

Bossel, H. (1998). Earth at a Crossroads. Cambridge: University Press.

Buckler, B. (1996) 'A learning process model to achieve continuous improvement and innovation', *The Learning Organization*, 3(3):31-9.

Burgelman, R.A. and Sayles, L.R. (1986) *Inside Corporate Innovation*, The Free Press, New York, NY.

Catalyst. (2000). *Cracking the glass ceiling*. NY: Catalyst.

Center for Women's Business Research. (1999, March 4) *Characteristics of women entrepreneurs worldwide*. Retrieved April 6, 2002, from http://www.nfwbo.org.

Chaganti, R. (1986). Management in women-owned enterprises. *Journal of Small Business Management*, 24(4), 19-29.

Chanda, Ashok and Kabra, Shilpa (2000) *'Human Resource Strategy-Architecture for Change,* Response Books, Sage Publications: New Delhi.

Chapman, J.A, Ferfolja, T. (2001) 'Fatal flaws: The acquisition of imperfect mental models and their use in hazardous situations', *Journal of Intellectual Capital,* 2 (4): 398–409.

Charmack, Thomas J. Lynham, Susan A. and Ruona, Wendy E. (2003) 'Critical Uncertainties Confronting Human Resource Development' *Advances in Developing Human Resources,* Vol. 5, No. 3 August.

Clothier, S. (2001). Cracking the glass ceiling in Europe. *The British Journal of Administrative Management,* 24(2), 21-29.

Collins, P.H. (2000). *Black feminist thought* (2nd ed.). NY: Routledge.

Day, G.S. (1990) *Mental Driven Strategy: Processes for Creating Value,* The Free Press, New York, NY.

Devetak, S. (2001) Obrobje v primezu globalizacije-problemi in dileme politike EU do jugovzhodne Evrope. Anthropos, 4/6, 68-76.

Dilworth, Lex (2003) 'Searching for the Future of HRD', *Advances in Developing Human Resources,* Vol.5, No. 3, August.

Dixon, Nancy M. (1990) 'Organisation Learning: A Review of Literature with Implications for HRD Professionals' *Human Resource Development Quarterly,* Vol. 3, No. 1.

Driskell, James E. and Salas, E. (1992) 'Collective Behaviour and Team Performance', *Human Factors,* Vol.34, No. 3.

Druckman, D. and Swets, J.A. (1988) (eds) *'Enhancing Human Performance: Issues, Theories and Techniques'* National Academy Press: Washington, DC.

E. Abraham, S. J. (1988) in Khandelwal, A. K. (ed.) *Human Resource Development in Banks*, Oxford and IBH Publishing Co., New Delhi.

Elliott, D., Smith, D. and McGuinness, M. (2000) 'Exploring The Failure To Learn: Crises and the Barriers to Learning', *Review of Business*, Fall/Winter, 21,3/4.

Fenwick, T. (1998). Women composing selves, seeking authenticity: A study of women's development in the workplace. *International Journal of Lifelong Education*, 17(3), 199-217.

Fenwick, T., & Hutton, S. (2000). Women crafting new work: The learning of women entrepreneurs. *Proceedings of the Adult Education Research Conference* (pp. 112- 120). Vancouver, BC: University of British Columbia.

Flax, J. (1989). Postmodernism and gender relations in feminist theory. In M. Malson, J. F. O' Barr, S. Westphal-Wihl, & M. Wyer (Eds.), *Feminist theory in practice and Process* (pp. 51-69). Chicago, IL: The University of Chicago Press.

Fletcher, J. K. (1999). *Disappearing acts: Gender, power, and relational practice at work.* Cambridge, MA: The MIT Press.

Garavan. T. (1997) 'The learning organization: a review and evaluation', *The Learning Organization* 4(1):18-29.

Garvin, D.A. (1993) 'Building a learning organisation', *Harvard Business Review*, 71, 78-91.

Gephart, M.A., Marsick, V.J., Van Buren, M.E and Spiro, M.S (1996) 'Learning Organisations Come Alive', *Training and Development*, Vol. 50, No. 12.

Globalisierung: Von der Vision zur Praxis. (1997) Zurich: Versus.

Gopalakrishnan, S. and Damanpour, F. (1992) 'Innovation research in economics, sociology, and technology management: a review and synthesis', *Proceedings of the Academy of Management*, 52, 488.

Grant, R.M.(1996) "Prospering in Dynamically Competitive Environments: Organizational Capability as Knowledge Creation." *Organization Science*, 7: 375-387.

Grant, R.M.(1996) Prospering in Dynamically Competitive Environments: Organizational Capability as Knowledge Creation. *Organization Science*, 7: 375-387.

Grundy, T.(1997) Human Resource Management- A Strategic Approach. *Long Range Planning*, Vol. 30, 4: 507-519.

Grundy, T.(1997) Human Resource Management- A Strategic Approach. *Long Range Planning*, Vol. 30, 4: 507-519.

Gupta, A.K. and Govindarajan, V., 1991, "*Knowledge flows and the structure of control within multinational corporations*", Academy of Management Review, 16.

Hanson, James A. (2001) *Indian Banking: Market Liberalization and the Pressures for Institutional and Market Framework Reform*, Working Paper No. 104, Stanford University.

Hiers, W. and Kuruvilla, S (1997) 'Globalisation and Industrial Relations in India' Paper for ILO Bangkok.

Hirschhorn, I. (1990) *The Workplace Within*, MIT Press, Boston, MA.

Honey, P. and Mumford, A. (1992), *The Manual of Learning Styles*, Peter Honey, Maidenhead.

Ibarra, H. (1993). Personal networks of women and minorities in management: A conceptual framework. *Academy of Management Review, 18*(1), 56-87.

Jackson, S.E. and Schuler, R.S. (1995) Understanding Human Resource in the context of Organizations and their

Environments. *Annual Review of Psychology*, 46: 237-264.

Jancar, D. (2004). Ura evropske resnice za Slovenijo. Delo, 3/1/2004, 13.

Jaques, E. (1953) 'On the dynamics of social structure', *Human Relations*, 6(1): 3-24.

Jarrett, M. and Kellner, K. (1996) 'Coping with uncertainty: a psychodynamic perspective on the work of top teams', *The Journal of Management Development*, 15(2): 54-68.

Kamau, D., McLean, G., & Ardishvilli, A. (1999). Women entrepreneurs: Maintaining business success through human resource development. *Human Resource Development Quarterly, 18*(2), 753-761.

Kamesam, Vepa (2003)The role of Quality Human Resource in Target Setting for Economic Growth. Address at a meeting organised by the Technology Information, Forecasting and Assessment (TIFAC), Centre of Relevance and Excellence (CORE), New Delhi, 25 July 2003.

Kamesam, Vepa (2003)The role of Quality Human Resource in Target Setting for Economic Growth. Address at a meeting organised by the Technology Information, Forecasting and Assessment (TIFAC), Centre of Relevance and Excellence (CORE), New Delhi, 25 July 2003.

Kanter, R.M., (1989) *When Giants Learn to Dance*, Unwin, London.

Kasl, E., Marsick, V.J. and Dechant, K (1997) 'Teams as Learners: A Research Based Model of Team Learning', *Journal of Applied Behavioural Science*, Vol. 33.

Kerka, S. (1993). *Women and entrepreneurship*. ERIC Clearinghouse on Adult, Career, and Vocational Education. Columbus, OH: Ohio State University.

Khandelwal, A. K. (ed.) (1988), *Human Resource Development in Commercial Banks*, Oxford and IBH Publishing Co: New Delhi.

Khandelwal, A.K. (1978), *Challenges in training in Banks*, Indian Journal of Training and Development, Vol. 8, No. 2, March - April, pp: 25-40.

Klein, M. (1975) *Envy and Gratitude and Other Works 1945-1963*, Virago, London.

Kogut, B. and Zander, U. (1992)Knowledge of the Firm, Combination Capabilities, and the Replication of Technology. *Organization Science*, 3. pp. 383-397.

Kogut, B. and Zander, U. (1992)Knowledge of the Firm, Combination Capabilities, and the Replication of Technology. *Organization Science*, 3. pp. 383-397.

Kolvereid, L., Shane, S., & Westhead, P. (1993). Is it equally difficult for female entrepreneurs to start businesses in all countries? *Journal of Small Business Management*, *31*(4), 42-53.

Kopac, M. (2004). Izgovori ne bodo pomagali. Delo, 3/1/2004, 16.

Kornhauser, A. (2004). Odprta vrata niso za zapeckarje. Delo, 3/1/2004, 14.

Kumar, Harish and Mishra, Alpana (2001) Role of IT in making HR Function Globally Competitive. People, Processes and Organisations-Emerging Realities. pp. 218-219.

Kuruvilla, S. (1999) 'Impact of Globalisation on Economies and IR/HR Systems—Theory and Evidence' in Sivananthiran, A. and VenkataRatnam, C.S. (eds.) *Globalisation and Labour Management Relations in South Asia*, Indian Labour Organisation Publications.

Larrain, J. (1994) 'The postmodern critique of ideology', *The Sociological Review*, 42 (2), 289-315.

Lynton, R and Pareek, Udai (1990), *Training for Development*, Kumarian Press: Connecticut, USA.

MA. Steiner, L. (1998) 'Organizational dilemmas as barriers to learning', *The Learning Organization*, 5 (4): 193 – 201.

MacDuffie, J.P., & Krafcik, J.F. (1992). *Integrating Technology and Human Resources for High Performance Manufacturing*, in T. A. Kochan and M. Useem, eds., Transforming Organizations. New York: Oxford University Press.

MacKeracher, D., & McFarland, J. (1993/1994). Learning working knowledge: Implications for training. *Women's Education des Femmes, 10*(3/4), 54-58.

Maheshwari, Amol and Jhajharia, Shweta (2001), *Private Sector Banks: Shaping Up*, Management Review, June.

Maira, Arun (2003), 'Setting the Course Amidst Turbulence', Background Papers, AIMA 30th National Management Convention, September 15 – 17.

Maira, Arun and Abraham, James (2003) 'Accelerating Organisational Learning' Background Papers, AIMA 30th National Management Convention, September 15 – 17.

Mamkootam, K. (1996) 'Globalisation, Restructuring and Industrial Relations in India', Paper presented at the Regional Meeting of the Asian Industrial Relations Association, Taipei, Taiwan, September.

Marquardt, Michael and Berger, Nancy O. (2003) 'The Future: Globalisation and New Roles for HRD', *Advances in Developing Human Resources*, Vol. 5, No. 3 August.

Marsick, V.J. and Watkins, K.E (1999), *Facilitating Learning in Organisations: Making Learning Count*, Gower: Aldershot, U.K.

Marsick, Victoria J and Watkins, Karen E. (2003) 'Demonstrating the Value of an Organisations Learning Culture: The

Dimensions of the Learning Organisation Questionnaire', *Advances in Developing Human Resources,* Vol. 5, No.2, May.

Martin H.P., Schumann H. (1997). Pasti globalizacije. Ljubljana: Co Libri.

Mayberry, M., & Rose, E.C. (Eds.). (1999). *Innovative feminist pedagogies in action.* NY: Routledge.

McClernon, T.R. and Swanson, R.A. (1995) 'Team Building: An Experimental Investigation of the Effects of Computer Based and Facilitator- Based Interventions on Work Groups', *Human Resource Development Quarterly,* Vol. 6, No. 1.

McGill, M.E., Slocum, J.W., Sei, D., (1992), 'Management practices in learning organizations', Organizational Dynamics, 21, 5-17.

Meen, D.E., Keough, M. (1992) 'Creating a learning organization', *The McKinsey Quarterly,* 1: 58-81.

Mencinger, J. (2004). Unija-zdruzba za cas sedmih debelih krav. Delo, 30/4/2004, 12.

Menzies, L. (1960) 'A case in the functioning of social system as a defence against anxiety', *Human Relations,* 13(2): 95-121.

Mintzberg, H., 1994, *The Rise and Fall of Strategic Planning,* The Free Press, New York, NY.

Mirza S. Saiyadain (1991) ' HRD- Currency Vs. Concept', *Indian Journal of Training and Development,* May-June.

Mitra, Monika,2003, *Banking on Backing,* Business Today, February, 2003 pp: 94-97

Mitroff, I., Pauchant, T., Finney M. and Pearson, C.(1989) 'Do (Some) Organizations Cause Their Own Crises? Culture Profiles of Crisis Prone versus Crisis Prepared Organizations', *Industrial Crisis Quarterly,* 3: 269-283.

Monappa, Arun (1997) Managing Human Resource. Mac Millan (India), New Delhi.

Moore, D. (2000). *Careerpreneurs.* Palo Alto, CA: Davies-Black Publishing.

Moore, D., & Buttner, H. (1997). *Moving beyond the glass ceiling.* Thousand Oaks, CA: Sage.

Mumford, A. (1996) *Creating a learning environment, Journal of Professional Human Resource Management*, 4, 26-30.

Munro, A., Holly, L., & Rainbird, H. (2000). My ladies aren't interested in learning: Managers, supervisors and the social context of learning. *International Review of Education, 46*(6), 515-528.

Naman, J.L., and Slevin, D.P. (1993) Entrepreneurship and the concept of fit: a model and empirical test', *Strategic Management Journal*, 14(2): 135-52.

Narasimham Committee (1998), *Report of the Committee on Banking Sector Reforms.*

Nelson, G. W. (1987). Information needs of female entrepreneurs. *Journal of Small Business Management, 25*(3), 38-44.

Orasanu, J. and Salas, E. (1993) 'Team Decision Making in Complex Environments' in Klein, G.A, Orasanu, J., Calderwood, R. and Zsambok, C.E (eds.) *Decision Making in Action: Models and Methods,* Norwood, NJ.

Ouchi, W.G. (1981) *Theory Z. How American Business Can Meet the Japanese Challenge,* Addison-Wesley, Reading.

Pascale, R. (1990) *Managing On The Edge,* Harmondsworth: Penguin. .

Pauchant, T.C. and Douville, R, (1993) 'Recent Research in Crisis Management: A Study of 24 Authors' Publications from 1986-1991', *Industrial and Environmental Crisis Quarterly*, 7 (1), 43-66.

Pauchant, T.C. and Mitroff, I (1992) *Transforming the Crisis-Prone Organization.* Preventing Individual Organizational and Environmental Tragedies, San Francisco: Jossey-Bass Publishers, 1992.

Pedler, M., Boydell, T. and Burgoyne, J. (1989) 'Towards the Learning Company', *Management Education and Development*, Vol. 20, No. 1.

Peters, T. J., & Waterman, R. H., Jr. (1982, 1986), *In search of excellence: Lessons from America's Best-Run Companies*, Harper & Row: New York; reprint, Warner Books: New York, 1986,

Polenec, A. (2004). Navajeni smo na konkurenco. Delo, 3/1/2004, 15.

Porter, M.(1985) Competitive Advantage: Creating and Sustaining Superior Performance. New York: Free Press.

Quinn, J.B., Anderson, P. and Finkelstein, S. (1996) 'Making the Most of the Best", *Harvard Business Review*, March-April.

Rao, T.V (1995) 'Changing Role of HRD in the Liberalized Economy' in Rao, T.V, Silveira, D.M, Srivastava, C.M and Vidyasagar, Rajesh (eds.) *HRD in the New Economic Environment*, Tata Mc Graw – Hill Publishing Company Ltd., New Delhi.

Rao, T.V. (1999) *HRD Audit*. Response Books, New Delhi.

Rao, T.V. (1999), *HRD in the New Economic Environment*, Tata Mc- Graw Hill: New Delhi.

Rao, T.V., Rao, R. and Yadav, T. (2001) A Study of HRD Concepts, Structure of HRD Departments and HRD Practices in India. *Vikalpa*, 26 (1): 49-63.

Rebula, A. (2004). Predvsem vprasanje samozavesti. Delo, 3/1/2004, 13-14.

Rosser, J.B. Jr, (1993) 'Belief: its role in economic thought and action', *The American Journal of Economics and Sociology*, 52(3): 355-69.

Rozier, C. (1995). Female entrepreneurs in a female-dominated health profession: An exploratory study. *Journal of Developmental Entrepreneurship*, 3(2), 149-163.

Russ-Eft, Darlene, Preskill, Hallie and Sleezer, Catherine (1997),'*Human Resource Development Review- Research and Implications*', Sage Publication: London.

Saxena, R.P. (1999) Information Technology as a Strategic Tool for Attaining Success in Global Environment. Paradigm, Vol. 3, No. 2, July-Dec. '95, pp. 95-104.

Schwartz, J. (1993) 'The paradox of ideology', *Canadian Journal of Philosophy*, 23(4): 543-75.

Shah, S.G. (1978), *How to make training in banking management*, CAPITAL, March, pp: 71-76.

Shah, Saiyadian and Sheth, N.R, (1984), *Human Resource Management in Banking Industry - Text and Cases*, South Asian Publishers.

Shukla, Madhukar (1997) '*Competing Through Knowledge-Building a Learning Organisation*', Response Books, Sage Publications, India.

SILS Industry Analysis Series (1997), *Banking Industry: Trends and Challenges*, March.

Silveira, D.M. (1988) '*Human Resource Development – The Indian Experience*, News India: Bombay.

Singh, Anup K. and Singh Romila (1995) Strategic Human Resource Management: A New Thrust for Indian Organisations. *MDI Management Journal*, Vol. 8, No. 1 (Jan. '95), pp. 39-52.

Singh, P.N. (1998) HRD Perspectives in the 21st Century. *The*

Indian Journal of Commerce, Vol. 51, No. 4, Oct.-Dec. 1998.

Slater, S.F. and Narver, J.C. (1995), Market orientation and the learning organization, *Journal of Marketing*, 59: 63-74.

Sodhi, J.S. (1993) 'New Economic Policies and their Impact on Industrial Relations,' *Indian Journal of Industrial Relations*, Vol. 29, No.1.

Som, A.(2002) Role of Human Resource Management in Organisational Development. Unpublished Doctoral dissertation Ahmedabad: IIM.

Sparrow, P.R. and Budhwar, P. S. ('97) Competition and Change: Mapping the Indian HRM Recipe against World -Wide Patterns. *Journal of World Business*, 32 (3): 224-242.

Spinder, D. (2000). Entrepreneurship-a learning process: The experiences of Asian female entrepreneurs and women in business. *Education and Training*, *42*(8/9), 445-452.

Stewart, T.A. (1997) *Intellectual Capital: The New Wealth of Organisations*. NC Currency Doubbledey, New York.

Stracher, G. (1999) 'Socially Responsible Enterprise Restructuring', in Enterprise Forum, Geneva.

Sun, P. and Scott, J.L. (2003) 'Exploring the divide - organizational learning and learning organization', *The Learning Organization*, 10(4):202-215.

Sykes, H.B., and Block, Z. (1989), 'Corporate venturing obstacles: sources and solutions', *Journal of Business Venturing*, 4(3): 159-67.

Tisdell, E. J. (1998). Poststructural feminist pedagogies: The possibilities and limitations of a feminist emancipatory adult learning theory and practice. *Adult Education Quarterly*, *48*(3), 139-156.

Toplak, C. (2003). Zdruzene drzave Evrope. Ljubljana: Fakulteta za druzbene vede.

Ulrich, D. and Lake, D. (1991) Organizational Capability: Creating Competitive Advantage. *Academy of Management Executive*, 7 (1): 77-92.

Venkataratnam, C.S and Verma, A. (1997) (eds.) *'Challenge of Change: Industrial Relations in Indian Industry'* Allied Publishers Pvt. Ltd., New Delhi.

Venkataratnam, C.S. (1999) (ed.) *'HRD for Adjustment at the Enterprise level,* Participants Manual, International Labour Organisation.

Verma, Madhurendra K. (2000) *'Nurturing Change Through Your Human Assets'*, Sage India.

Vince, Russ (2003) 'The Future Practice of HRD', *Human Resource Development International,* Vol. 6, No. 4, December.

Vreg, F. Globalizacija in elektronska demokracija. Teorija in praksa, 38, 1.

Wajcman, J. (1998). *Managing like a man: Women and men in corporate management.* University Park, PA: The Pennsylvania State University Press.

Watkins, K.E. and Marsick, V. (1992).' Building the Learning Organisation: A New Role of Human Resource Developers' *Studies in Continuing Education,* Vol. 14, No.2.

Watson, G., (1993) 'The fuss about ideology', *The Wilson Quarterly*, 16(1): 130-36.

Wells, S. J. (1998). *Women entrepreneurs: Developing leadership for success.* NY: Garland.

Woodman, R.W., Sawyer, J.L., Griffin, R.W. (1993), 'Towards a theory of organizational creativity', *Academy of Management Review*, 18(2): 293-321

Wright, P.M. and McMahan, G.C. (1992) Theoretical Perspectives for Strategic Human Resource Management. *Journal of Management*, 18 (2): 295-320.

Yang, Baiyin (2003) 'Identifying Valid and Reliable Measures for Dimensions of a Learning Culture', *Advances in Developing Human Resources,* Vol. 5, No. 2.

Yorks, Lyle and Sauquet, Alfonso (2003), 'Team Learning and National Culture: Framing the Issues' *Advances in Developing Human Resources,* Vol. 5, No. 1, February.

Zeks, B. (2004). Veè ambicije, prosim. Delo, 3/1/2004, 17.

INDEX

A

Academy of Human Resource Development, 2
AHRD, 4
Alternative Flow Patterns, 184
American Society for Training Directors, 2
ASTD, 4
Automation, 91

B

Blue-collar and white-collar workers, 151
Boggus, J.L. 197

C

Career,
- authority and control, 175
- choices, 150
- Development, 15
- opportunity information, 172
- renewal, 179

Civil Rights Act of 1964, 162
Collaboration, 105
Concept of Manpower Information Systems, 130-146
Concepts of Human Resource Planning 81-103
Communication, 220
Concurrent validity, 167
Consultants, 111
Content validity, 167
Coping with Changed Conditions, 107

D

Dagenham, 211
Diversification, 107
Downward and lateral career mobility, 178

E

Early reservations, 84
Early retirement, 178
Education and training, 94
Education programs, 172
EEOC, 153
EETPU, 224
Elton Mayo, 2
Employee Career Development, 169
Employee Effectiveness, 161
Employee task forces, 166
Employment Act of 1967, 177
Empowerment, 33
Entrepreneurship, 33

European legislation, 190
Executive Council, 98
Exposure, 117
Extraordinary maturity, 166

F

Fawley Blue Book, 208
Flow Policies/Systems Designing, 191
Ford Motor Company, 208, 222, 227

G

General Systems Theory, 5
Golden WOnder, 201
Green Paper, 225
Gutteridge and Otte, 15

H

Hawthorne Studies, 2
HRD Function, 109
HRD: Training and Development, 113-129
HRM outcomes, 191
Human Beings as Capital, 84
Human Capital Theory, 5
Human Resource Development, 1
A Philosophical Interpretation, 35-80
Human Resource Flow Management, 147-196
Human Resource, 85, 88
Human Resources Development Planning, 104-112
Human Resource Management, 248-270

I

India, China and Bangladesh, 101
Institute of Applied Manpower Research, 99
Institutional Theory, 5
Integrated Child Development Scheme, 99
Integrated Human Resources Development, 83
Internal Flow Management, 158
Issues in Training and Employment, 24
Issues in Training and Employment, 24-34

J

Jaguar, 218
Japanese workers, 151
Job posting, 175
Job Requirements, 120
Joining up, 158

K

Knowledge economy, 18
Knowledge management, 17
Knowledge workers, 18

L

Labour, 85
Lawson, 225
Leadership and motivation, 220
Learning, 7, 17
Legal, 181
Line Manager(s), 11, 111
Long, 223

Low Input Sustainable Agriculture, 101

M

Management, 182
Managing Flow Perspective, 148
Managing Human Resources in Practice, 197-236
Managing Inflow, 156
Manpower, 85, 86
Planning, 89
Maslow, 35
McLagan, 8
McLean and McLean, 7
Megginson, 7
Mental aptitude, 41

N

National Health Service, 199
National Vocational Qualifications, 3
NEDO, 199

O

One-man-one job, 28
Openness and Risk-Taking, 105
OPQ Test, 218
Organisational Development, 16
Organisational Perspective, 154
Out Placement, 32
Outflow Management, 176

P

Participation in a training program, 170
Personnel development specialists, 175
Personnel specialists, 163
Perspective Building, 33
Perspective, 181
Peter Principle, 160
Planning Commission, 97, 98
Policies, Systems and Practices, 155
Postwar planning, 90
predictive validity, 167
Preparing HRD Plan, 108
Proactivity, 105
Psychological contract, 158

Q

QC, 226
Quotas mandate, 169

R

Recruiting Effectiveness Criteria, 157
Recruitment decisions, 156
Recruitment and selection, 216
Resource-Based Theory, 5
Robert Conken, 177

S

SHRD, 1, 9
Standing Committees on Research Programmes, 98
Stewart, 8
Strategic decisions, 151
Strategic Human Resource Development (SHRD), 8
Strategic Human Resource Development, 1-23

Sustainable Development, 101
Systematic Training, 117

T

Team management, 29
Technological change, 90
Technology mission, 99
Terminations, 177
Top management group, 192
Trainers, 115
Training and Development, 14, 113
Training of Management Trainees, 121
Training, 6, 29
  types Activities, 30
Trevor, 219
Trust and Authenticity, 105

U

United States, 153
University Forum for HRD, 3, 8

V

Velocity of Personnel Flow, 159
Vestibule school, 117

W

Walton, 3, 9
War Manpower Commission, 86
Weitzman (Prof.), 225
White, 219
Wickens, 129
Women and Child Development, 98
Workrom training in, 118
World War II, 86, 90, 91